A Defense *of* Dignity

NOTRE DAME STUDIES IN MEDICAL ETHICS

O. Carter Snead, series editor

The purpose of the Notre Dame Studies in Medical Ethics series, sponsored by the Notre Dame Center for Ethics and Culture, is to publish works that specifically address contemporary issues in the field of medicine. The aim is to foster a systematic and rational discussion of medical ethical problems grounded in Catholic intellectual tradition and moral vision.

A Defense *of* Dignity

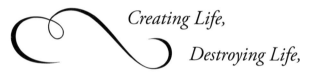

Creating Life,
Destroying Life,
and Protecting the Rights of Conscience

CHRISTOPHER KACZOR

University of Notre Dame Press
Notre Dame, Indiana

Dedicated to Elizabeth,

Who Made My Life Rich

Contents

Acknowledgments

Though each has been revised, the collected essays that constitute this book first appeared elsewhere. I am grateful to the respective publishers for their permission to make use of this material: "The Ethics of Ectopic Pregnancy: A Critical Reconsideration of Salpingostomy and Methotrexate," *Linacre Quarterly* (August 2009): 265–82; "Embryo Adoption and the Artificial Uterus," in *The Ethics of Embryo Adoption and the Catholic Tradition,* ed. Sarah-Vaughan Brakman (London: Springer, August 2007), 313–28, with kind permission of Springer Science and Business Media B.V; and "Organ Donations After Cardiac Death," *The Ethics of Organ Donation,* ed. Steve Jensen (Washington, DC: Catholic University of America Press, 2011), 95–113.

Several of the essays appeared online at *Public Discourse: Ethics, Law, and the Common Good,* the online journal of the Witherspoon Institute of Princeton, NJ: "The Importance of Dignity: A Reply to Steven Pinker," http://www.thepublicdiscourse.com/2012/01/4540/; "Let's Talk about Abortion: A Response to Dennis O'Brien," http://www.thepublic discourse.com/2011/09/3998/; "Equal Rights for All, Born and Unborn," http://www.thepublicdiscourse.com/2011/04/2310/; and "Abortion, Conscience, and Doctors," http://www.thepublicdiscourse.com/2010/10/1922/.

I am also grateful for the permission to use "Faith, Reason, and Physician-Assisted Suicide," *Christian Bioethics* 4.2 (1998): 183–201; and "Conscientious Objection and Health Care: A Reply to Bernard Dickens," *Christian Bioethics* 18.1 (2012): 59–71.

Chapter 1 is reprinted with permission from Philosophy and Theology Notes, *National Catholic Bioethics Quarterly* 10.1 (Spring 2010): 175–81, © 2010 National Catholic Bioethics Center. Chapter 2 is reprinted with permission from Philosophy and Theology Notes, *National Catholic Bioethics Quarterly* 10.4 (Winter 2010): 799–805, © 2010 National Catholic Bioethics Center. Chapter 3 is reprinted with permission from Philosophy and Theology Notes, *National Catholic Bioethics Quarterly* 10.3 (Fall 2010): 395–401, © 2010 National Catholic Bioethics Center. Chapter 4 is reprinted with permission from Philosophy and Theology Notes, *National Catholic Bioethics Quarterly* 9.3 (Fall 2009): 591–97, © 2009 National Catholic Bioethics Center. Chapter 7 is reprinted with permission from Philosophy and Theology Notes, *National Catholic Bioethics Quarterly* 11.4 (Winter 2011): 789–94, © 2011 National Catholic Bioethics Center. Chapter 8 is reprinted with permission from Philosophy and Theology Notes, *National Catholic Bioethics Quarterly* 11.3 (Autumn 2011): 579–85, © 2011 National Catholic Bioethics Center. Chapter 10 is reprinted with permission from Philosophy and Theology Notes, *National Catholic Bioethics Quarterly* 7.3 (Autumn 2007): 595–600, © 2007 National Catholic Bioethics Center. Chapter 11 is reprinted with permission from Philosophy and Theology Notes, *National Catholic Bioethics Quarterly* 9.4 (Winter 2009): 775–81, © 2009 National Catholic Bioethics Center. Chapter 12 is reprinted with permission from Philosophy and Theology Notes, *National Catholic Bioethics Quarterly* 11.2 (Spring 2011): 163–68, © 2011 National Catholic Bioethics Center.

I am also indebted to my research assistants Nicole Antonopoulos and Mariele Courtois.

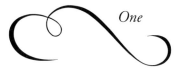

One

Introduction

The subject of human dignity has received a fair bit of attention. Both the report of the President's Council on Bioethics, *Human Dignity and Bioethics,* and the Vatican declaration *Dignitas Personae* have highlighted the idea of human dignity in the public eye while they have also raised important and difficult questions.[1] "What exactly is "dignity"? What is "human dignity"? Do human beings have it innately, or only conditionally? Should human dignity matter to us? In these introductory remarks, I will suggest answers to these questions.

The collection of essays that constitute this book examine ethical issues related to human dignity. The chapters fall into four groupings. Chapters 1–2 treat the dignity of the human person and consider arguments from advocates of animal rights that it is unjust to accord dignity to all human beings while declining to extend the same rights to non-human animals. Chapters 3–8 address the procreation of human life (including issues such as "procreative beneficence") and the immediate beginning of life (including issues such as ectopic pregnancy and fetal surgery). Chapters 9–11 focus on the end of life (including the issues of

treatment of PVS patients, physician-assisted suicide, and organ donation after cardiac death). The last two chapters attempt to defend the dignity of health care professionals who seek to serve others by following the
dictates of their consciences. As a presupposition to treating all of these
issues, it is important to ask whether the very concept of "dignity" has a
useful place in contemporary ethical debates.

A number of recent works have analyzed human dignity.[2] Perhaps
the most polemical contribution is the article "The Stupidity of Dignity"
by Steven Pinker, who argues against the usefulness of dignity as a central
principle in bioethics.[3] In addition to criticizing the ambiguity of the
term "dignity," Pinker sees three problems with making use of dignity as
a principle of bioethics, namely its relativity, its fungibility, and its potential for harm. He therefore rejects the concept of "human dignity" in arguments about bioethics and proposes to rely solely on the notion of
"autonomy." Pinker first illustrates the problematic relativity of the concept of dignity:

> First, *dignity is relative.* One doesn't have to be a scientific or moral
> relativist to notice that ascriptions of dignity vary radically with the
> time, place, and beholder. In olden days, a glimpse of stocking was
> looked on as something shocking. We chuckle at the photographs of
> Victorians in starched collars and wool suits hiking in the woods on
> a sweltering day, or at the Brahmins and patriarchs of countless so-
> cieties who consider it beneath their dignity to pick up a dish or play
> with a child.[4]

Pinker fails, however, to note that the concept of autonomy is also relative. The importance of autonomy in contemporary discourse can be
traced historically to the philosophy of Immanuel Kant, who described it
as the self-given law of practical reason shared universally by all rational
beings. Kant himself considered it always contrary to autonomy to commit suicide for any reason, to lie with any intention in any circumstance,
or to have sexual intercourse outside of marriage. Many contemporary
philosophers, however, enlist autonomy as a justification for conclusions
contrary to those drawn by Kant. If dignity cannot work as a central prin-

ciple in bioethics because it is relative historically, autonomy cannot work as a central principle in bioethics for the same reason.

Pinker offers the fungibility of dignity as his second rationale for dropping dignity from the vocabulary of bioethics. He writes:

> Second, *dignity is fungible*. The [President's] Council and [the] Vatican treat dignity as a sacred value, never to be compromised. In fact, every one of us voluntarily and repeatedly relinquishes dignity for other goods in life. Getting out of a small car is undignified. Having sex is undignified. Doffing your belt and spread-eagling to allow a security guard to slide a wand up your crotch is undignified. Most pointedly, modern medicine is a gantlet of indignities. Most readers of this article have undergone a pelvic or rectal examination, and many have had the pleasure of a colonoscopy as well. We repeatedly vote with our feet (and other body parts) that dignity is a trivial value, well worth trading off for life, health, and safety.[5]

Here again, Pinker fails to notice that autonomy is also fungible. Soldiers give up some autonomy when they enlist for military service. Employees give up autonomy when they sign contracts agreeing to perform certain services and to refrain from activities that constitute conflicts of interest. Police officers, FBI agents, and politicians relinquish autonomy when they swear to enforce the laws of our nation. Lawyers and psychologists give up autonomy by preserving confidentiality. Day care workers, parents of young children, and school teachers likewise diminish their autonomy in order to serve the young. Patients give up all their autonomy—at least temporarily—when agreeing to lose consciousness during surgery. Do the actions of these people reveal that autonomy is a trivial value, well worth trading for money, public order, confidentiality, the rearing of children, or health? Obviously, these considerations do not justify the conclusion that autonomy is a term that is not suitable for use in bioethical debates, so neither should similar considerations lead to the exclusion of the term dignity.

Pinker offers his third rationale for ditching dignity as an ethical value:

Third, *dignity can be harmful.* In her comments on the *Dignity* volume, Jean Bethke Elshtain rhetorically asked, "Has anything good ever come from denying or constricting human dignity?" The answer is an emphatic "yes." Every sashed and be-medaled despot reviewing his troops from a lofty platform seeks to command respect through ostentatious displays of dignity. Political and religious repressions are often rationalized as a defense of the dignity of a state, leader, or creed: Just think of the Salman Rushdie fatwa, the Danish cartoon riots, or the British schoolteacher in Sudan who faced flogging and a lynch mob because her class named a teddy bear Mohammed. Indeed, totalitarianism is often the imposition of a leader's conception of dignity on a population, such as the identical uniforms in Maoist China or the burqas of the Taliban.[6]

Pinker fails here, as well, to note that autonomy, too, can be harmful to society and to individuals. Desmond Hatchett exercised his sexual autonomy by fathering twenty-one children with eleven different women before the age of thirty.[7] Similarly, Nadya Suleman, unemployed and unmarried, used in vitro fertilization to add eight more babies to her other six young children at home. Drug abusers exercise their autonomy to harm themselves physically and mentally. Politicians regularly exercise their autonomy to implement unreasonable taxes, unfair laws, and unjust wars for their own political gain. Indeed, misuse of autonomy arguably causes much more harm than misuse of dignity.

These *tu quoque* responses to Pinker are less than satisfactory insofar as serious questions can and should be raised about the definition, role, and importance of the concept of dignity in bioethics. Echoing Ruth Macklin, Pinker highlights the ambiguous ways in which the term "dignity" has been used in bioethical discussions. The ambiguity of the term is an important issue that deserves serious consideration, something that Pinker himself fails to offer.[8] He also fails to notice that "autonomy" itself carries many meanings—autonomy as any self-initiated action, autonomy as informed consent, autonomy as the law of practical reason shared by all rational beings, autonomy as control, autonomy as authenticity.[9] The difficulty of ambiguous use of words is not unique to the term "dignity." Indeed, there is no term that cannot be used ambiguously. Admittedly "dignity," at this stage of common usage, seems even more prone to ambiguous usage than "autonomy," but that is not sufficient reason to dismiss it entirely or to prejudicially abandon attempts at disambiguation.

How, then, ought we to define dignity? Daniel P. Sulmasy, OFM, has distinguished three ways in which the term is used in contemporary ethical discourse: dignity as attributed, dignity as intrinsic worth, and dignity as flourishing.[10] Attributed dignity is the worth human beings confer on others or on themselves. For example, the dignity of a university president dressed in doctoral robes leading a solemn academic procession might be contrasted to the lack of dignity of the drunken bum sleeping face down on the beach. Attributed dignity comes in degrees and is at issue in many of the examples raised by Pinker.

Attributed dignity is to be distinguished from intrinsic dignity. Intrinsic dignity is described by Sulmasy, who writes:

> By intrinsic dignity, I mean that worth or value that people have simply because they are human, not by virtue of any social standing, ability to evoke admiration, or any particular set of talents, skills, or powers. Intrinsic dignity is the value that human beings have simply by virtue of the fact that they are human beings. Thus we say that racism is an offense against human dignity. Used this way, dignity designates a value not conferred or created by human choices, individual or collective, but is prior to human attribution. Kant's notion of dignity is intrinsic.[11]

The beach bum and the university president both have intrinsic dignity as human persons that cannot be lost as long as they live. Intrinsic dignity is an essential characteristic of being human and does not vary according to race, religion, age, sex, birth, nationality, or handicap, or so I'll argue later.

Dignity as flourishing consists in the excellence of a human life consistent with, and expressive of, intrinsic dignity. It accords with dignity as flourishing that human beings should be treated with respect, and violates human dignity as flourishing to mutilate and torture someone.

This simple, threefold disambiguation resolves the alleged contradiction of meaning claimed by Pinker. Slavery and degradation are morally wrong because they undermine someone's dignity as flourishing. However, nothing you can do to a person, including enslaving or degrading him, can take away his intrinsic dignity. Dignity as attributed reflects excellence, striving, and conscience, such that only some people achieve it by dint of effort and character. Everyone, no matter how lazy, evil, or mentally impaired, has intrinsic dignity in full measure, but not dignity as flourishing or as attributed. Once the three senses of dignity are distinguished, the concerns about ambiguity expressed by Pinker no longer obtain.

These three disambiguated senses of dignity will be seen to inform the different parts of this book. Some of its questions concern intrinsic dignity, in particular the issue of who has intrinsic dignity. Some concern dignity as attributed, for example, when someone treats another person as if they have no intrinsic worth. A number of questions bear on immoral actions that violate a person's dignity as flourishing. Unless otherwise noted, when I refer to "dignity" without further qualification, I usually mean intrinsic dignity rather than dignity as attributed or dignity as flourishing.

Even if we can successfully disambiguate the term, why is the principle of dignity important? Why should we employ it at all? My answer is that the concept of dignity does a better job than the concept of autonomy in describing and accounting for the intrinsic value of every human being. We are valuable not simply because of our choices, nor do we have value only while we are exercising our autonomy. We have value when we cannot choose due to temporary or even permanent disability. In his 2009 Tanner Lectures, "Dignity, Rank, and Rights," Jeremy Waldron pointed out that in ancient times dignity was accorded in particular to persons regarded as royalty or nobility. Noble persons were accorded rights, privileges, and immunities in keeping with their elevated rank. At its best, says Waldron, contemporary society does not reduce the noble but rather elevates the commoner, making every single human person equal in rank (with its corresponding privileges and immunities) to the duke or the lady. Although these ideals are often imperfectly realized in our society, Waldron has a point when he writes, "we are not like a society which has eschewed all talk of caste; we are like a caste society with just one caste (and a very high caste at that): every man a Brahmin. Every man a duke, every woman a queen, everyone entitled to the sort of deference and consideration, everyone's person and body sacrosanct in the way that nobles were entitled to deference or in the way that an assault upon the body or the person of a king was regarded as a sacrilege."[12] The term "dignity" captures the elevated status of the human person, every human person, better than most, if not all, other terms.

Pinker fails to see that autonomy cannot serve to justify the basic ethical principle he proposes: "Because all humans have the same minimum capacity to suffer, prosper, reason, and choose, no human has the right to impinge on the life, body, or freedom of another."[13] If autonomy were the basis for our rights (rather than the capacities named by Pinker), then in addition to denying rights to unborn human beings, Pinker would also have to exclude the severely mentally handicapped, the senile elderly, and newborns. Pinker's principle that all human beings share the same basic moral immunity from harm is the same in extension, if not also in meaning, as the principle that all human beings have a shared, basic dignity. Unfortunately, Pinker practices an ethics of exclusion according to which some human beings are disposable material for the use of other human beings.

Do we have any reason for ascribing intrinsic dignity to all human beings? There are a number of ways to argue for the proposition that all human beings are endowed with intrinsic dignity and certain inalienable rights. The first is that our dignity should be based on who we are, the kind of being that we are, rather than on how we are functioning in the moment. Dignity should be based on our membership in the human family, rather than on any particular performative activity. Our functioning, whether it be understood in terms of our ability to experience pleasure and pain, our consciousness, or our intelligence, comes in many degrees. If we think that our individual value as persons is based on a degreed characteristic, an "accident" in terms of Aristotelian metaphysics, then we cannot secure equal basic dignity and equal basic rights for all persons. We should therefore base our fundamental ethical judgments on the substantial identity of who we are rather than on any accidental degreed quality. Because all human beings are endowed with the same nature as members of the same kind—*Homo sapiens*—they all share equally basic rights and dignity.

Don Marquis sees a problem with this argument:

> Kaczor argues that the right to life must be based upon endowment, not performance. What people are capable of *doing* comes in degrees. This is incompatible with our commitment to human equality. Therefore, the right to life must be based on our endowment, on the genetics that we have in common with all other human beings . . . . [O]ne wonders why the right to life cannot be an equal right that one obtains by meeting some performance threshold, just as all students who pass their junior year[s] in high school have the equal right to enroll for their senior year[s], whether they passed their junior year[s] with flying colors or barely eked out passing grades.[14]

Important differences exist, however, between meeting the performance threshold for academic advancement and various performance accounts of personhood. First, in standards for grade advancement, there ought to be a nonarbitrary pedagogical relationship between what is to be learned in one grade and suitable preparedness for the next. By contrast, as I argued in *The Ethics of Abortion: Women's Rights, Human Life, and the Question of Justice,* there is no rational basis for determining which performance characteristic grants personhood to human beings (self-awareness, reasoning ability, sentience?) and what degree of that characteristic gives moral worth.

Second, if a degreed characteristic grants moral status, then it would seem to follow that the more you have of the valuable characteristic, the more valuable you would be. The junior who barely passed and the junior who earned a 4.0 both count equally as seniors, but they do not count equally in terms of their academic achievement as students. Likewise, performance-threshold accounts of personhood can establish that two normal adults both count as persons, but given vast human inequalities in degreed qualities (self-awareness, intelligence, etc.), such accounts cannot establish that any two particular individual adults have *equal moral worth* as persons, and hence equal rights.

Third, threshold accounts arbitrarily exclude some humans from having rights but include others. Take any degreed property that allegedly gives someone a right to live, such as self-awareness, sentience, or intelligence. Intelligence comes in many degrees, and the threshold view holds that once a human being reaches a certain degree of intelligence then he or she has a right to life. Due to mental illness and cognitive disabilities of various kinds, the degree of intelligence among individual human beings varies widely along a continuum. Xavier is an adult human being who just barely achieves the threshold degree of intelligence, but because he "barely" or "only just" clears the threshold, he has a right not to be intentionally killed. Yolanda, another adult human being, has only a fractionally lower degree of intelligence than Xavier, but because of this tiny difference she does not have a right not to be intentionally killed. The difference in intelligence between Xavier and Yolanda is infinitesimally small; yet the threshold view holds that we may treat them in radically different ways. This is arbitrary. A trivial difference between the two cannot justify a radical difference in treatment. By contrast, advancing a student who barely passed and requiring the failed student to repeat a grade is not treating the students in such radically different ways. Both continue their education, albeit at different grade levels. We should, therefore, reject threshold views of basic human rights, even if the threshold views makes sense in other contexts where less radical consequences follow.

Another way of justifying human dignity is in terms of the orientation of all human beings towards rationality and freedom. Unlike other species, human flourishing is achieved by means of and partially constituted by human freedom and reason rather than mere instinct. The flourishing of human beings, but not non-human animals, necessarily involves freedom and rationality. The moral goods are also partially constituted by human reason and freedom. Because all of us as human beings are ordered to these moral goods, human beings are also moral agents in a passive sense; that is, they should be respected as moral agents when they are on the receiving ends of actions, even when they are not at that time or even at any time actually performing actions as moral agents.

I presuppose that it is wrong for other agents to intentionally inhibit your flourishing in any significant way. This is true not simply for you individually but universally for all others who share a flourishing like yours: an ordering to goods such as friendship, knowing the truth, and moral integrity. Because all human beings share the same basic way of flourishing, and because it is wrong (aside from just punishments) to intentionally inhibit this flourishing in you or anyone whose flourishing is like yours, it is wrong to intentionally inhibit the flourishing of any human being. If this judgment is correct, then all human beings—sharing as they do in having flourishing-like-yours—have basic moral status and dignity.

Marquis critiques this way of justifying the thesis that all human beings should be accorded moral status:

> Kaczor's strongest argument appeals to what he describes as the orientation of all human beings toward freedom and reason. The virtue of this move is that it gets our values into the account of the basis for our rights. The trouble with this move is that either this orientation is entirely a matter of the genetics that make us members of the human species or it is not. On the one hand, if it is just a matter of our human genetics, then, perhaps, it may yield the equality of all human beings. The trouble is that some individuals who are genetically enough like us to be counted as humans, such as the irreversibly unconscious, are not capable of freedom and reason.[15]

It is true that the irreversibly unconscious are not capable of freedom and reason, but my argument was not based on capability or potentiality either immediate or remote. Capability for freedom and reason is not equivalent, in meaning or extension, to orientation towards freedom and reason. The orientation towards freedom and reason is not abolished in irreversibly unconscious human beings, though this orientation is frustrated by disease or injury. Indeed, it is precisely the orientation to freedom and reason of all human beings that makes it so tragic when injured human beings cannot pursue distinctively human goals. The illiterate man is tragically deprived; the illiterate ape is not. This concept of flourishing plays a similar role in my justification of human dignity and universal human rights as the "future-like-ours" plays in Marquis's own justly famous essay on abortion.[16] I am disappointed that Marquis did not notice the parallels between his view and my own view (both of which are non-species specific) in the following passage of the book Marquis was reviewing. I wrote:

> Aside from just punishments, it is a violation of your rights when someone intentionally undermines your flourishing or what is necessary for your flourishing. To kill you is to undermine . . . your flourishing because being alive is necessary for you to flourish and is itself partially constitutive of your flourishing, so it is wrong to kill you. This is true not simply of you as an individual but of all others whose flourishing is similar to yours. So, it is wrong to kill any other being who shares flourishing-like-yours. This norm then would exclude the intentional killing of all innocent human beings and any other being sharing flourishing-like-yours.[17]

My account secures the right to life of irreversibly comatose human beings whose flourishing is like ours, but whose flourishing is greatly compromised by their unfortunate disabilities. If this argument is correct, then it is incumbent upon people of good will to aid, rather than harm, human beings with such disabilities. This choice is relevant for issues to be discussed later in this book including physician-assisted suicide, organ donation, and provision of nourishment to those who are permanently unconscious.

This argument brings us to the overcommitment objection to universal human rights and dignity. Marquis writes:

> The claim that all human beings have a serious right to life seems to imply that a human being who is in an irreversibly unconscious state, such as an anencephalic child or someone who has experienced severe trauma to her brain or is totally brain dead, has a serious right to life. It certainly seems counterintuitive to suppose that it would be as wrong to end the life of such a human being as it would be to end the life of you or me.[18]

I do believe that human beings who are permanently unconscious retain their intrinsic dignity and basic human rights. "Total brain death" is a different matter, because *if* (it remains a disputed matter) brain death truly is death, then there is no human being in such a case, but rather only a corpse with residual activities resembling life. Such entities, being already dead ex hypothesi, cannot (as a matter of metaphysics rather than ethics) have a right to live.

Brain death aside, Marquis is correct that killing you or me is worse than killing a permanently unconscious human being, but one need not deny equal basic human rights to come to this conclusion. In addition to violating the right to life shared equally by all innocent human beings, killing us also thwarts our future plans and makes it impossible for us to fulfill our duties. These additional circumstances add to the depravity of intentionally killing the innocent, but are missing in cases of human beings who are permanently unconscious. In a similar way, an ordinary person has the same right to life as an important politician has, yet political assassination is worse than garden-variety murder. Assassinating a president or prime minister is worse than murdering an ordinary person due to the greater political and social repercussions of the killing, yet the right to life of every innocent person is equal.

Marquis provides no argument to justify his assertion that permanently unconscious human beings should not be respected, but merely appeals to an allegedly shared intuition that permanently unconscious humans do not have an equal right not to be intentionally killed as you or I do. So, let's change the case. A woman has a right not to have sexual intercourse without her consent. It is obvious, therefore, that a hospital janitor who rapes an unconscious woman does wrong, whatever the duration of her lack of consciousness. But if a permanently unconscious woman retains her right not to be raped, then her neurological condition does not result in the loss of her basic human rights, so she would also retain her right not to be intentionally killed, a right she shares with her brothers and sisters who are in utero or who are in the last stages of life.

Marquis's critique of the case for universal human dignity does not succeed. It is certainly not, as Marquis describes it, "the Catholic view" in any sectarian sense. It can and has been endorsed by people of good will of a variety of faith traditions and of no faith tradition. It is the view endorsed by the 1948 United Nations Declaration of Human Rights: "Everyone is entitled to all the rights and freedoms set forth in this Declaration, without distinction of any kind, such as race, colour, sex, language, religion, political or other opinion, national or social origin, property, birth or other status." Unfortunately, political, legal, and social recognition for all human beings remain more aspirations than achievements in the contemporary world, especially those at the beginning or end of life.

Another way of justifying the intrinsic dignity of all human beings is proposed by S. Matthew Liao. In Liao's view, all human beings have a right to live in virtue of their genetic disposition to moral agency. Of course, not all human beings are constantly acting as moral agents, but all human beings have the genetic basis for moral agency. This genetic basis is species-neutral, so there may or may not be other beings that also have dignity and rights. This genetic basis is a sufficient condition for dignity, so other beings may have rights on other bases.[19]

After noting the ambiguities in the ways in which human dignity is used in bioethical debates—for example, as a premise to argue both for and against physician-assisted suicide, an issue we will consider later in this work—Jukka Varelius suggests a problem with Liao's view:

> It might be maintained that all human beings have rational nature by virtue of having the genetic structure of a rational being. That could work in the case of the human dignity of otherwise normal persons in minimally conscious state. However, the genetic constitution of some non-human beings, such as bonobos, can be more similar to the typical genetic structure of humans, the paradigm rational beings, than is that of genetically defected [sic] humans.[20]

Proposing another dilemma, Varelius goes on to argue that having the genetic structure of a rational being does not grant dignity. If only minor alterations in the genetic structure are permitted, then many defective humans do not have dignity because they have major genetic defects. In this case, not all human beings have dignity. But if major alterations in genetic structure are permitted, then non-human animals would also have rational nature and so non-human animals would have dignity. In this case, defenders of dignity would have to embrace a strong commitment to animals rights, which they characteristically do not want to do (even though it is not logically excluded simply by being committed to the dignity of all human beings).

Liao has provided a basis for an answer to this argument by escaping the first horn of the dilemma:

> The genetic defects that we are likely to encounter in these severely defective human beings are not defects in the genetic basis for moral agency but at best defects that undermine the development for moral agency. For example, consider Phenylketonuria (PKU), Tay-Sachs, Sandhoff Disease and a whole cluster of about 7000 other kinds of genetic disorders, which are caused by the mutation of a gene. The gene is typically necessary for producing a certain protein or enzyme, which is then needed to change certain chemicals to other chemicals or to carry substances from one place to another. Mental retardation and other defects are typically caused by abnormal build-ups of certain amino acids that become toxic to the brain and other tissues, because the cell is unable to process these amino acids owing to the mutation. But with treatment of a low enzyme diet as soon as possible in the neonatal age, normal growth and cognitive development can be expected in many cases. For our purpose, this shows that the brain tissue has initially developed normally and would have continued to do so except for the abnormal build up of the amino acids. Therefore, following the distinction between genetic defects that make up an attribute and genetic defects that undermine the development of the attribute, single gene defects seem to be cases of the latter rather than the former. Given this, one can say that human beings who have these kinds of genetic defects most likely have the genetic basis for moral agency.[21]

If Liao is correct, even human beings with severe genetic defects that undermine the development of a particular attribute would still have the genetic basis for rationality, and this would also separate them from higher order primates. Varelius's argument rests on a misunderstanding of the nature of genetic defects.

One more objection to human dignity raised by Varelius and also echoed by various neo-Darwinians is that, "in light of evolution, it can be argued, there are no real or important differences between such species as, for example, humans and great apes."[22]

Do we differentiate human beings and great apes on the basis of differences that are not "real" but merely figments of our imagination? On the contrary, there are objective, empirically verifiable differences between the species in terms of appearance, behavior, reproductive possibilities, and genetic constitution. Are these differences unimportant? One can admit a shared origin of all species, yet also recognize that, from this shared origin, species have developed that are really and substantially different. In some cases, the real and substantial difference is more radical (bacteria and human beings) and in other cases less radical (great apes and human beings), but it is in every case substantial. If the human species is substantially different from others species, it is not unfair to treat them in ways that accord with this difference.[23]

That human beings differ from all other species, and that this difference is ethically germane, is recognized even by some advocates of neo-Darwinism. Ben Dixon, for example, offers a "Darwin-approved argument for human dignity [that] centers on the idea that humans are the only creatures capable of creating, maintaining, and expanding institutions for moral reasons."[24] He argues that it is a difference in kind and not just in degree between human beings and non-human animals. If Dixon is correct, then we have yet another basis for human dignity, aside from the Christian and Kantian foundations already widely proposed and the genetic basis suggested in Liao's article mentioned earlier.

Yet advocates of animal rights among others deny any important ethical distinction between human beings and animals. Do human beings alone have intrinsic dignity? Why shouldn't animals, particularly those with high intelligence such as dolphins and great apes, also be accorded dignity? Are the differences between human beings and non-human animals morally relevant? It is to the important question of animal rights to which we now turn our attention.

Two

Are All Species Equal in Dignity?

Almost everyone agrees that *some* human beings have dignity, basic rights, or moral worth, but whether any non-human animals have dignity, basic rights, or moral worth remains a matter of great debate. The debate over animal rights involves many different questions. Is eating meat morally permissible?[1] Can hunting be justified?[2] Do sentient animals deserve greater consideration than non-sentient human beings? This chapter focuses on a single aspect of the debate: Is species membership relevant to ethical judgment? Advocates for animal rights reject what they call "speciesism." "[Peter] Singer defines 'speciesism' as 'a prejudice or attitude of bias in favor of the interests of members of one's own species and against those of members of other species.' Speciesism, like sexism and racism, is a prejudice involving a preference for one's own kind, based on a shared characteristic that in itself has no moral relevance."[3]

Varelius raises the objection that human dignity is inherently unjust towards other species. He says that "it could be maintained that granting all and only members of the human species special dignity is speciesism and, accordingly, morally on a par with such isms as sexism and racism."[4]

According to Varelius, we should therefore reject granting dignity to all human beings as inherently unfair to non-humans.

This often-repeated charge against human dignity rests on two confusions. The first is merely linguistic. Racism and sexism are wrong, but we cannot simply add "ism" to some class of characteristics to create a morally illegitimate point of demarcation. After all, advocates for animal rights characteristically endorse either sentientism (valuing sentient beings over non-sentient beings) or autonomism (valuing autonomous beings over non-autonomous beings). To simply assert that denying dignity on the basis of species is as morally dubious as denying dignity on the basis of race or sex is to beg the question—which is precisely whether non-human animals are equal or not in dignity to human beings.

Second, even if speciesism is ethically problematic, a commitment to the dignity of all human beings does not involve a denial of dignity to any other class of non-human beings simply because they are not human. Those who defend the dignity of all human beings need not believe, and characteristically do not believe, that *only* humans have dignity. A Catholic view, for example, holds that God the Father, God the Son, and God the Holy Spirit, as well as angels, are also persons with dignity. Even aside from religious beliefs, it is possible that there very well may be many other beings in the universe, such as intelligent aliens, who have a rational nature and therefore have dignity even if they are non-human. Of course, such beings would not have *human* dignity because they are not human, but they would have dignity. The belief that *all* human beings have dignity does not imply a commitment to the view that *only* human beings have dignity. In other words, the question of whether or not we are morally obligated to recognize "animal rights" is simply not answered by a commitment to the equal, intrinsic dignity of all human beings.[5] To be a human being is a sufficient, but not a necessary, condition for moral worth. This leaves open the possibility that there are many other beings of moral worth who are not human.

Before considering the arguments for and against speciesism, it is important to point out that Singer's definition of speciesism begs the question. The words "prejudice" and "bias," like the words "cruelty" or "merciless," are not merely descriptive but also negatively evaluative in a moral sense. Prejudice and bias are wrong, so speciesism is already—solely in virtue of Singer's stipulated definition rather than any reasoned justification—also wrong. Thus, Singer's definition begs the question. This weakness in Singer's definition can be seen when the context is not animal rights but the rights of the human fetus. I propose to be against "birthism," which I define as a prejudice or bias in favor of the interest of those who are born against those who are not yet born. Birthism, like sexism and racism, is a prejudice involving a preference for one's own kind, those already outside the uterus, based on a shared characteristic that in itself has no moral relevance.[6] Surely, to be against "birthism" is merely another way of stating that I am in favor of fetal rights or that I am opposed to abortion. Thus, invoking "birthism" or "speciesism" does not settle the issue, but rather implicitly endorses one side of a debated question. Precisely at issue is whether birthism or speciesism really is like racism or sexism, and rhyming neologisms do not settle the ethical question. Let me propose a non-question-begging definition of speciesism: the belief that species membership is ethically relevant.

In Dale Jamieson's view, speciesism has two important features. "First, what is of primary moral relevance is individuals and the properties they instantiate, not the fact that they may be members of various collectives or kinds. Thus, for purposes of morality, properties such as being a member of the Lions Club or a citizen of the United States are not in themselves of central moral importance. Second, the individual characteristics that are morally relevant are not properties such as species, race and gender, but rather characteristics such as sentience, the capacity for desire and self-consciousness."[7] Both features merit comment.

If we take "morally relevant" to mean necessary for basic rights and dignity, then it would seem that being members of some particular collectives or kinds is morally irrelevant. No one's basic moral rights should hinge on whether or not they are members of the Lions Club or citizens of the United States. However, examples such as these do not show that membership in particular kinds is always irrelevant. Presumably, only those in the class of living beings can have a right to life, only those in the class of sentient beings can have a right not to be tortured, and only those in the class of intelligent beings can have a right to education. Indeed, when formulating ethical norms or rules of public policy, it is necessary—if our formulations are to make use of collective nouns and reflect ethical universalizability—to appeal to groups of some kind.

Secondly, there is reason to believe that characteristics such as sentience, the capacity for desire, and self-consciousness are not necessary for basic moral status.[8] These characteristics come in various degrees, so if ethical status is based on the degree of possession of such characteristics, then we have to hold that even normal adult human persons do not have equal rights. Furthermore, these characteristics exclude some beings (such as handicapped newborns) that virtually everyone accepts as persons with basic rights.

In another article, Peter Singer presents "a graduated view of the moral status of humans and nonhuman animals."[9] An opposing view is represented by Catholic tradition: "Pope John Paul II and those who accept his position on this issue think not only that all humans are equal to each other but also that they are far superior to nonhuman animals. The philosophical problem is whether we can justify that view."[10]

Putting aside philosophy for a moment, Singer presents a number of theological justifications for the Christian view that human beings have a greater moral worth than non-human animals, rejecting each: "1. We are made in the image of God, and animals are not. 2. God gave us dominion over animals. 3. We have immortal souls, and animals do not." We can add to these theological justifications some considerations not explicitly raised by Singer but relevant at least for Christian theists. According to Christian view, Jesus is sinless. But Jesus commanded Peter to catch fish (Luke 5:4) and himself ate fish (Luke 24:41–43). If Christians are right that Jesus did not sin, eating fish cannot be intrinsically evil because Jesus both eats fish and commands others to facilitate eating fish. The Passover ritual requires the slaughter of a lamb (Exodus 12:5–10). The Gospel of Luke states, "Jesus sent Peter and John, saying, 'Go and prepare the Passover for us, that we may eat it'" (Luke 22:8). In telling his disciples to prepare for the Passover ritual (which would be formal cooperation in evil if eating meat was wrong), Jesus authorizes the slaughter of a lamb for human consumption and then eats lamb meat himself (Mark 14:18). Both the teachings and actions of Jesus point to the intrinsic dignity of all human beings regardless of their health status (the leper), social status (the tax collector), or religion and sex (the Samaritan woman). Therefore, the actions and teachings of Jesus suggest that human persons have a basic equality and a greater status than animals, at least greater than that of lambs and fish.

Of course, as an atheist, Singer rejects the theological justifications he considers. Interestingly, he gives no arguments to justify his rejection; he just asserts without explanation that they are mistaken. He therefore gives theists and Christians no reason to question, let alone reject, the theological justifications mentioned for making a moral distinction between human beings and non-human animals. It makes no more sense for a Christian to presuppose an atheistic perspective in considering the question of animal rights than for an atheist to presuppose a Christian perspective.

Singer also asserts, again without justification, that even if the theological justifications mentioned were true, they would provide no basis for law or public policy in a pluralistic society. This assertion is also problematic. Even if religious grounds are not a sound basis for public policy (here the opposing arguments of Richard John Neuhaus among many others are important to keep in mind),[11] these religious arguments still may provide a sound basis for religious people to hold the view—as a matter of personal ethics—that all human beings are equal and that all human beings have greater moral worth than all non-human animals.

A second ground for preferring human beings over animals considered by Singer does not appeal to revelation. Singer summarizes his view of Kant's defense of human dignity: "Kant's argument for why human beings are ends-in-themselves is that they are autonomous beings, which, in terms of Kantian philosophy, means that they are capable of reasoning. Note that Kant goes from defending the value of autonomy or self-consciousness to maintaining that 'man' is the end. If we really take his argument seriously it means that human beings who are not self-conscious—because perhaps they are so profoundly mentally retarded that they lack self-consciousness or self awareness—are also merely means to an end, that end being autonomous or self-conscious beings."[12] So, by Singer's understanding of Kant, if a human being lacks self-consciousness, then that human being does not have to be respected as an end-in-itself and may be treated simply as a means.

Obviously, neither Kant nor any other reasonable person thinks that actual self-consciousness is necessary for basic moral worth. If this were so, then whenever people are in surgery or otherwise pass out, they lose their moral status only to gain it back upon waking. Singer is correct that autonomy is central to Kantian ethics, but it is central not because it is the ground for human dignity. Rather, autonomy is important for Kant as a consequence of Kant's strict requirement that we should do what is in accordance with duty, motivated by duty (*die pflichtmäßige Handlung aus Pflicht*).[13] For Kant, if emotional inclinations such as desire for rewards or fear of punishments dictate which action an agent performs, then the agent's action has an improper motivation and the act has no moral worth. If we are to act rightly, then our actions must be autonomous, motivated by the self-given law of reason.

For Kant, all human beings, due to their rational nature (but not necessarily their rational functioning), have inherent dignity. Kant would view the step towards evaluating human worth in terms of functionality instead of ontology as a confusion of persons and things. Things are evaluated according to how they function, and the price of a thing is determined by human desire for the well or poorly functioning thing. Beings of a rational nature have dignity but no price because they are the possible seat of the only thing that is good without qualification: the good will. The value of a being with rational nature follows from its very nature rather than from its function as healthy or ill, young or old, beautiful or ugly, or even valued by others or not valued by others.

The best historical treatment of Kant's views on these matters is probably Patrick Kain's "Kant's Defense of Human Moral Status." Kain points out: "Personhood and responsibility do not entail that each person acts or has acted, or that each is always able to act; it only entails that *when* or *if* a person does act, she may be held responsible for her actions."[14] He continues:

Within Kant's theory, existence as a living member of the human species is taken as a sufficient indication of basic moral status because membership in that species indicates the presence, in a perceptible being, of the status-grounding predisposition to personality. Since, according to Kant's Formula of Humanity, it is impermissible to treat any being with dignity as a mere means, Kant's position entails that it is impermissible to fail to treat any human organism as an end-in-itself, which seems to entail a strong, though defeasible, presumption against, for example, the intentional killing of any human organism at any stage of its development.[15]

Anyone interested in Kant's thoughts on these matters should carefully study Kain's magisterial article, which corrects misinterpretations of Kant like those propounded by Singer.

Singer rounds out his reflections on various grounds for believing in human superiority over animals by treating social contract views.[16] Singer also rejects this justification because newborns cannot enter into contracts of any kind. Logi Gunnarsson tries to shore up this difficulty, "There is an important difference between the great apes in nature and severely disabled infants, a difference that does not concern their intrinsic abilities but rather their relationship to humans: Only the latter are dependent on humans for their well-being. The dependency of a being on a human being is a source of a duty for human beings different in kind from the intrinsic abilities of the great apes that give rise to duties toward them."[17] The implicit premise seems to be that we have a moral duty to provide for other human beings that which is necessary for their flourishing.

Eva Feder Kittay presents an interesting argument for this premise:

> If McMahan, [Singer], and others acknowledge the special relationship that is constituted by parenthood, and if they can grant that the parent of a child with the severe cognitive impairments has a deeper and morally and objectively more significant relationship with that child than does a pet owner with his beloved pet, then I believe that a number of implications suggest that the recognition of the child as possessing moral personhood must follow. I as a parent have obligations to fulfill toward any child of mine. Following Sarah Ruddick, we can say that what a child "demands" of its parent is to assure that the child's life is protected, that the child's development and growth are fostered, and, as I have already pointed out, that the child can find social acceptance. Now, no parent with a child of typical capacities can do this in a vacuum. All parents need access to certain

resources to fulfill their obligations to their child, ones that are at least partially supplied by the larger society. Every parent needs schools and other social institutions to ensure that her child can develop her capacities, whatever those capacities may be. Every parent needs to work with both the child and the social world that the child enters to ensure that the child will grow into a member who is granted respect and who can develop a sense of self-respect. No child is simply the parent's own private matter. If McMahan and Singer claim to honor my relationship to my child and to grant its moral significance, then they cannot with any consistency grant the means to fulfill parental obligations to one parent and deny them to another parent based on some set of features of the child, for these are what all parents need to fulfill their ethical responsibilities to their children regardless of their capacities and needs."[18]

This argument secures the rights of handicapped newborns but does not justify giving similar rights to great apes. Thus, there may be a contractarian justification for treating all human beings in ways that we do not treat animals.

After reviewing a theological, a Kantian, and a contractarian justification for according moral immunities to human beings but not animals, Singer reasons: "Hence we have to conclude that the standard ethical view that we find expressed in the statement by John Paul II—the view that all human beings, irrespective of their cognitive abilities, have equal moral status, and that this status is superior to the moral status of the most intelligent nonhuman animals—cannot be defended."[19] Even if Singer had refuted the religious, Kantian, and contractarian arguments for basic human equality and superiority over animals, his conclusion is still a non sequitur. Surely, we have no reason to think that there are only three ways to defend the idea that all human beings ought to be accorded equal rights above non-human animals. Conspicuous by absence are the Aristotelian-Thomistic philosophical arguments that all human beings have equal basic moral status superior to non-human animals.[20]

Singer makes the point—using extensive empirical evidence—that some animals (great apes, dogs, gray parrots) have greater cognitive abilities than some human beings (the profoundly mentally handicapped, the newborn).[21] He assumes, but never justifies through argumentation, that greater or lesser moral status is correlated with greater or lesser cognitive ability. If we accept this view, then it is true that some human beings are not morally equal in basic dignity to some animals, but it is also true that, based on this view, we cannot secure the basic equality of human persons whose cognitive abilities vary widely. Surely, a college student does not have greater basic moral worth than a kindergartener, despite having greater cognitive ability. Certainly, our basic moral status does not shift many times over the course of our lives. We lose or gain cognitive abilities based on which drug is in our system (Ritalin vs. marijuana), but our dignity does not shift episodically as various chemicals alter our brains. We have strong reason to reject the idea that greater or lesser moral status is correlated with greater or lesser cognitive ability.

We also have good reason to reject the view that speciesism is akin to racism or sexism. Accepting the wrongfulness of speciesism commits one to implications that are deeply counterintuitive. First, if speciesism is wrong, then we should not grant special protections to animals that are members of endangered species because being a member of a particular species is morally irrelevant. Secondly, if speciesism is wrong, then we should also refrain from helping animals of a particular species that are suffering from overpopulation because that, too, would involve treating some animals differently than others in an ethically significant way based on species membership.[22] Singer's and Jamieson's arguments against speciesism suggest that we should also forcibly prevent animals from killing each other because we often forcibly prevent some human beings from killing other human beings. Finally, imagine that I rush into a burning building and I have time to save only one of two beings at the same level of consciousness. I find a one-year-old girl and nearby her the family dog, both passed out from smoke inhalation. "As Singer notes in *Animal Liberation,* everything else being equal, someone who rejects speciesism should be morally indifferent between a human and a dog who are at the same level of consciousness."[23] If speciesism is wrong, then I should just flip a coin to decide whether to save the girl or the dog. This is absurd. Much remains to be discussed in terms of the subject of animal rights, but the arguments advanced against speciesism by Singer and Jamieson fail to justify their conclusions.

If we recognize that all human beings should be accorded respect and treated in accordance with their intrinsic dignity, then the question naturally arises about how this equality ought to inform social practices. Does basic human equality entail that all human choices are deserving of respect? If all human beings should be unconditionally accorded the rights, privileges, and moral immunities which once were enjoyed only by nobles or ladies of stature, then how does this inform our ethical practices, particularly with respect to creating human life? It is to this topic which we now turn.

Three

Equal Dignity and Equal Access to Fertility Treatments

If all human beings have intrinsic dignity, this dignity extends to the very beginnings of human life and the procreation of human life itself. For this reason and others, the ethical response to infertility, including the risks of IVF to women and children,[1] remains a topic of much discussion.[2] An important contribution was published in 2009 by the Ethics Committee of the American Society for Reproductive Medicine (ASRM), entitled, "Access to fertility treatment by gays, lesbians, and unmarried persons." The ASRM report addresses the question of whether those working in health care should assist individuals in reproducing, regardless of marital status or sexual orientation. Obviously, if the conclusions reached thus far in this book are correct, unmarried people as well as gays and lesbians share equal basic dignity with every other human person and therefore also have equal basic rights. Based in part on this recognition, the summary conclusions of the ASRM report include the following, "There is no persuasive evidence that children are harmed or disadvantaged solely by being reared by single parents, unmarried parents, or gay and lesbian parents. . . . Programs should treat all requests for assisted reproduction equally without regard to marital status or sexual orientation."[3] Not only may health care workers assist in the request to reproduce, the report asserts that they must assist. "Although professional autonomy in deciding who to treat is also an important value, we believe that there is an ethical obligation, and in some states a legal duty, to treat all persons equally, regardless of their marital status or sexual orientation."[4]

What justifies these conclusions? The report mentions shifting public standards such as increasing trends in society away from reproduction by married, opposite-sex couples and a greater acceptance of homosexuality. The committee also breaks down the ethical debate into three main points. First, the ASRM holds that unmarried persons as well as gays and lesbians have reproductive interests. Secondly, the committee believes that the welfare of children is not impeded by being reared in a nontraditional family. Finally, the report curtails the personal autonomy and conscience rights of health care workers in favor of a "duty not to discriminate on the basis of marital status or sexual orientation."[5] Each of these points merits further investigation.

The invocation of "societal standards" is remarkably inconsistent throughout the report. For example, shifts in social acceptance of single parenthood are noted as evidence in favor of assisting unmarried individuals in reproducing, but societal views of same-sex marriage are simply ignored as evidence against assisting same-sex couples in reproducing. As of 2009, when the ASRM report appeared, in thirty-one different states— including left-leaning California—same-sex marriage was put to a vote of the people, and in all thirty-one states a majority of the people voted against same-sex marriage. At the time it was written, the drafters of the report were not justified as claiming social acceptance of same-sex marriage. Neither voting nor polling indicated that society viewed opposite-sex couples and same-sex couples as equivalent. The ASRM committee provides no evidence whatsoever that "society" approves of treating all requests for assistance in reproduction equally regardless of marital status or sexual orientation. Polls have found that society in general disapproves of adoption by same-sex couples of children already in existence and in need of parents, so how much more would society likely disapprove of creating a child specifically for same-sex couples? Even if polling showed that most people support adoption by same-sex couples, the views of the majority do not determine what is ethically acceptable. The ASRM report, however, proceeds as if this were the case, at least when the majority supports the conclusions to which the committee is predisposed. When public opinion does not support the conclusions to which the committee is predisposed, public opinion is ignored.

The committee asserts, "Given the importance to individuals of having children, there is no sound basis for denying to single persons and gays and lesbians the same rights to reproduce that other individuals enjoy."[6] Since the state does not criminalize single parenthood or constitutionally ban assisted reproduction by homosexuals or the unmarried, "moral condemnation of homosexuality or single parenthood is not itself an acceptable basis for limiting child rearing or reproduction."[7]

There are, however, no such things as "rights to reproduce." This would amount to the right to have a child; but children—like all other human beings—are not property to which other persons could have rights. The lack of such a "right" applies equally to unmarried and married, to straight, gay, and lesbian persons. People do have "parental rights" because they have parental duties—duties which only come into existence along with the existence of the child. No one—married or unmarried, heterosexual, or homosexual—has the "right" to a child. Children, like all human beings, are not property to which one could have a legal or moral right. One could posit, however, a right of access to fertility care which would permit questions about who has and does not have this right.

Further, it simply does not follow that because some practice is legal, then a health-care practitioner cannot use a moral condemnation of the practice as a reason not to assist in a procedure. Termination of a pregnancy during the ninth month simply because the fetus is female is legal in the United States, but even the least generous protection of conscience allows health care workers to decline to perform abortions in this situation. Physician-assisted suicide is legal in Oregon and Washington, but virtually everyone agrees that doctors ought not to be forced to help kill their patients. Capital punishment is constitutionally legal in the United States, but who would force physicians opposed to the death penalty to participate in it? The report's move from the premise of legality to the conclusion that the legality warrants a civil duty to assist is a non sequitur.

The ASRM asserts that: "The evidence to date, however, cannot reasonably be interpreted to support such fears," as that a child will risk adverse outcomes if not reared by a married mother and father. "Those clinicians who will not treat single females, for example, may believe that fertility treatment should be restricted to married couples, that treatment should be for the infertile only, or that children need a father and a 'normal upbringing.'"[8]

No evidence is cited by the committee to support the claim that being reared by a single parent does not endanger the well-being of children. Indeed, vast evidence suggests that children reared by single parents, including children reared by cohabiting parents, risk adverse effects with respect to mental health, physical well-being, academic achievement, emotional problems, incarceration, abuse of drugs and alcohol, and failure to establish lasting relationships as adults. The evidence is summarized in a number of publications including *Why Marriage Matters: Twenty-Six Conclusions from the Social Sciences.* The evidence is overwhelming that raising offspring outside of marriage endangers the well-being of children. For example, in comparison with unmarried couples, *Why Marriage Matters* notes that children reared by their married biological parents have "better physical health, on average, than do children in other family forms. . . . Parental marriage is associated with a sharply lower risk of infant mortality."[9] Single and cohabiting parents put the well-being of their children at risk. As David Popenoe and Barbara Dafoe Whitehead note, "Cohabiting parents break up at a much higher rate than married parents, and the effects of breakup can be devastating and often long lasting. Moreover, children living in cohabiting unions with stepfathers or mother's boyfriends are at higher risk of sexual abuse and physical violence, including lethal violence, than are children living with married biological parents."[10] The conclusion that children fare better—physically, socially, legally, educationally, and psychologically—when reared by their married parents is well established in the social sciences.

Given the overwhelming evidence strongly pointing to the disadvantages for children of being reared by a single parent (of whatever orientation), let us turn now to another issue reared by the committee, namely fertility treatment for gays and lesbians. Do same-sex couples provide the same benefits to children as opposite-sex couples? We cannot simply assume that because children do better when reared by their married opposite-sex parents, they will do equally well being reared by a same-sex couple. There are significant innate, genetic, biological differences between men and women and therefore between mothers and fathers.[11] In every case, children reared by same-sex couples are always deprived of either their own father or their own mother. In a fascinating discussion of why it would be wrong to conceive a child in order to place the child for adoption, Bernard G. Prusak argues that parents have imperfect duties to provide for their own children in ways that only they can.[12] Prusak provides a framework for coming to the following conclusion: to create children knowing that they will not have the special care of their own mother (or father) is to fail in an imperfect obligation to the child.

In contrast to their treatment of single parenthood, the ASRM committee does provide some support for the claim that children reared by same-sex couples do not have a higher rate of social or psychological problems. The ASRM notes the conclusion of an American Psychological Association task force which held, "Research suggests that sexual identities (including gender identity, gender role behavior, and sexual orientation) develop in much the same way among children of lesbian mothers as they do among children of heterosexual parents. . . . Studies of other aspects of personal development (including personality, self-concept, and conduct) similarly reveal few differences between children of lesbian mothers and heterosexual parents."[13] The report admits that less evidence is available for the outcomes of children reared by gay men, but it also suggests that the limited evidence indicates that gay men are better fathers than straight men.

The evidence is not as unequivocal as the ASRM summary leads one to believe. For example, in his article "The Potential Impact of Homosexual Parenting on Children," Lynn Wardle in the *University of Illinois Law Review* argues that systemic bias among researchers in favor of liberal social views of homosexuality distorts their research on the issue.[14] He notes, for instance, that the subjects in these studies are often self-selected, rather than randomly selected; the control groups sometimes consist of single parents, rather than opposite-sex couples; the sample sizes are too small to be statistically reliable; the studies rely on retrospective data and self-reporting; and the research does not control for education, employment, health, and other relevant factors. He also points out that we have few longitudinal studies of the long-term effects of same-sex parenting. Finally, Wardle notes:

> The "social desirability" bias taints the studies of homosexual parenting. Both researchers and respondents perceive that within society, or at least the subgroup of society with which they identify, it is deemed desirable, progressive, and enlightened to support one particular outcome—in this case, that homosexual parenting is just as good as heterosexual parenting. This insight influences the research design and analysis, as well as the data gathered—the responses.[15]

These flaws in the data used by advocates of same-sex parenting are recognized even by self-described "pro-gay" scholars such as Judith Stacey and Timothy Biblarz, who are both strong advocates of same-sex marriage and childrearing by same-sex couples. In their 2001 *American Sociological Review* article, "(How) Does the Sexual Orientation of Parents Matter?" they write:

> Because researchers lack reliable data on the number and location of lesbigay parents with children in the general population, there are no studies of child development based on random, representative samples of such families. Most studies rely on small-scale, snowball and convenience samples drawn primarily from personal and community networks and agencies. Most research to date has been conducted on white lesbian mothers, who are comparatively educated, mature, and reside in relatively progressive urban centers, most often in California or the Northeastern states. . . . Most studies simply rely on a parent's sexual self-identity at the time of the study, which contributes unwittingly to the racial, ethnicity, and class imbalance of the populations studied.[16]

In contrast, none of these flaws taint the research about single parenthood and cohabitation mentioned earlier.

Even if we were to ignore the methodological flaws in the research on same-sex parenting and take the existing findings as sound social science, the ASRM summary of findings is still misleading. A number of studies have found significant differences between children reared in heterosexual marriage and those reared by same-sex couples. Stacey and Biblarz argue that these differences have a positive or simply different influence on children, but it is possible to view some of these differences as detrimental. For example, Stacey and Biblarz note that "Tasker and Golombok (1997) also report some fascinating findings on the number of sexual partners children report having had between puberty and young adulthood. Relative to their counterparts with heterosexual parents, the adolescent and young adult girls reared by lesbian mothers appear to have been more sexually adventurous and less chaste."[17] Interestingly, the same study found that boys reared by lesbians were less sexually adventurous as men, but since females are more at risk from "sexually adventurous" behavior, this is a small comfort. Although not available at the time of the drafting of the ASRM report, more recent social science research has called into question the idea that same-sex couples and opposite-sex couples are equally likely to have favorable outcomes when raising children.[18]

Many people believe that homosexuality is a genetic trait, like eye color, determined from birth and unrelated to environmental factors. However, studies of monozytogic twins, who share the same genes and uterine environment, have found that identical twins do not always share the same sexual orientation.[19] Because identical twins do not always share the same sexual orientation, environmental factors such as parenting play a role in the development of sexual orientation. Stacey and Biblarz note, "64 percent (14 of 22) of the young adults reared by lesbian mothers report having considered a same-sex relationship (in the past, now, or in the future), compared with only 17 percent (3 of 18) of those reared by heterosexual mothers."[20] Similar effects appear to be found in other research: "[One] study [on gay fathers and their adult sons] also provides evidence of a moderate degree of parent-to-child transmission of sexual orientation."[21]

Some people point to sociological evidence indicating that opposite-sex couples on the whole behave differently than same-sex couples and that these differences are relevant to the raising of children. According to these studies, opposite-sex couples tend to have relationships of longer duration, tend more towards monogamy and sexual fidelity, and tend to have less violence than do same-sex couples.[22] If this evidence about differences between same-sex couples and opposite-sex married couples is correct, then assisting a same-sex couple in conception places that child at greater risk for adverse consequences than assisting an opposite-sex, married couple. Children are likely to benefit more from being reared in family forms that tend to be more enduring, monogamous, and nonviolent.

Finally, the ASRM report asserts: "As a matter of ethics, we believe that the ethical duty to treat persons with equal respect requires that fertility programs treat single persons and gay and lesbian couples equally to heterosexual married couples in determining which services to provide."[23] This conclusion is a non sequitur. Equal respect for the dignity of persons does not entail equal respect for *every* decision a person makes, let alone a duty to assist in every decision a person makes. Every person, regardless of sexual orientation, marital status, or other circumstance, deserves equal respect of their basic rights such as life and liberty; this entails a duty for each individual not to intentionally kill or enslave any person. Equal respect does not entail a doctor's duty to do whatever a patient requests. Imagine a knock on the door of a fertility clinic. It is a single mother of fourteen children via assisted reproduction, whose oldest child is seven. She requests another round of IVF with eight more embryos to be implanted at once. According to the argument advanced by the ASRM, a physician not only *may* but *must* help her to have more children, lest the physician not respect her decision and her equality with other persons.[24] This is absurd. There is also generally a moral and legal duty not to discriminate according to age, but it would be obviously wrong to assist an eighty-five-year-old woman in reproduction.[25]

The recognition of the equal dignity of all persons does not mean that all persons have an equal right to access to fertility treatments. The physician is not at the absolute command of the patient. Dictates of conscience apply, particularly when the well-being of not only the patient but also an actual or potential child is involved. The definition, role, and importance of conscience are all undeveloped in the ASRM report. Respect for the wishes of the prospective parents is underscored, but respect for the physician's conscience is ignored. How can we know whether the demands of conscience trump the requests of a patient for assistance in reproduction unless we know something more about what conscience is and why conscience can make moral claims upon us? The report does not contribute to our understanding of this important question, a topic I will return to later.

In sum, ASRM's "Access to Fertility Treatment by Gays, Lesbians, and Unmarried Persons" does not provide sound guidance for decisions about assisting persons with infertility problems. The committee report relies on false premises, reasons invalidly, ignores well-known and abundant contrary evidence, leads to absurd conclusions, and fails to address the central question about the relationship of conscience to providing fertility treatment. The recognition of the equal dignity of all persons does not mean that all persons have an equal right to access to fertility treatments.

The questions surrounding fertility treatments are not limited to the ones discussed in this chapter. Scholars have also raised concerns about whether there is an obligation to use fertility treatments in such as way as to maximize the likelihood of a child having a good life. The next chapter treats the debate about "procreative beneficence."

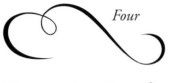

Four

Procreative Beneficence

After the Second World War, eugenics earned a nearly universal bad name and was widely viewed as incompatible with human dignity, but recent ethicists have sought to rehabilitate eugenics in a non-racist, non-totalitarian form. Do we have a duty to choose children whose genetic endowments would predispose them to have the best life? Julian Savulescu is perhaps the most articulate and prolific defender of an affirmative answer. With Guy Kahane, Savulescu defines the Principle of Procreative Beneficence (PB) as follows:

> If couples (or single reproducers) have decided to have a child, and selection is possible, then they have a significant moral reason to select the child, of the possible children they could have, whose life can be expected, in light of the relevant available information, to go best or at least not worse than any of the others.[1]

Although in the future, sperm sorting may be able to accomplish PB prior to conception, PB can now be accomplished in two ways: either by use of prenatal testing during pregnancy (amniocentesis, ultrasound, etc.)

followed by abortion of those deemed unacceptable or through the use of in vitro fertilization (IVF) and preimplantation genetic diagnosis (PGD). In this essay, I focus on the second form of PB, which makes use of IVF and PGD.[2] Savulescu and Kahane support PB by appeal to a more general principle that to make ethically good procreative choices, parents must consider the prospective well-being of the potential child. "When we make decisions, the option we should choose is the one which maximizes expected value. In the case of selection and reproductive decision making, the outcome of interest should be how well a new person's whole life goes, that is, well-being. PB thus states that we have reason to select the child who is *expected* to have the most advantaged life."[3] According to this view, we should accept PB because of the more general obligation of parents to maximize the chances that their child will have a good life.

Do advocates for PB, including Savulescu and Kahane, accept the full implications of this general principle? Do they consistently apply it in evaluating reproductive choices? Upon consideration, it indeed turns out that this more general principle—that potential parents should procreate with the greatest expected well-being of their possible children in mind—leads to the rejection of PB.

First, there is evidence to suggest that the use of IVF itself increases the likelihood that the child will have serious birth defects. One "study suggests that children born by IVF have an increased risk of developing cerebral problems, in particular cerebral paralysis."[4] Another study concludes, "Children conceived with the use of 'Intracytoplasmic Sperm Injection' (ICSI) or IVF run a double risk of presenting a greater defect at birth in relation to the general population."[5] The Centers for Disease Control and Prevention reported that birth defects, including heart wall problems, may be two to four times more likely for children conceived through assisted reproductive technology than for children conceived naturally.[6] The long-term epigenetic risks of IVF are simply not yet known.

Of course, any given child conceived by IVF may be free from such birth defects, and thankfully most of them are. However, the general principle justifying PB is that parents should choose for their potential children the life that would maximize well-being, taking into account the likelihood that their choices will actually further that end. Since IVF itself does not maximize likely well-being, the general principle justifying PB leads to a rejection of IVF and therefore also a rejection of PB which necessarily involves IVF.

Even if using IVF did not increase the likelihood of disability, Savulescu and Kahane do not consistently apply the principle that prospective parents should maximize the expected well-being of their potential children. They hold that "if couples (*or single reproducers*) have decided to have a child . . . , then they have a significant moral reason to select the child, of the possible children they could have, whose life can be expected, in light of the relevant available information, to go best or at least not worse than any of the others."[7] If Savulescu and Kahane consistently applied their principle, they would support reproduction only by married couples. Children conceived and reared by married parents—rather than single parents, cohabiting parents, or divorced parents—have lower rates of poverty, better relationships with their own parents, better physical health, greater success in school, lower rates of mental illness and psychological distress, lower rates of substance abuse, less trouble with the law, lower rates of being abused physically or sexually, lower rates of teen pregnancy, higher stability in their own intimate relationships as adults, and lower likelihood of death by accident, addiction, or suicide.[8]

Therefore, the general principle that parents should give their children the best chance at the best life also implies that parents have a moral obligation to conceive and rear children only within marriage. If we have a moral obligation to maximize the likely well-being of children, then this reproductive moral obligation excludes single reproducers as well as cohabitating couples from reproducing because children reproduced and reared in these circumstances have significantly less expected well-being than those reproduced and reared by a married mother and father. Unless advocates of PB are willing to endorse the moral obligation of marriage as a prerequisite for ethically acceptable procreation, they need to find a new general principle to justify PB. If "reproductive autonomy" (itself not a morally unproblematic concept) overrides the obligation to procreate and rear children only in marriage, then "reproductive autonomy" should also generally override PB.

Ultimately, Savulescu and Kahane justify the duty to maximize the likely well-being of children on the basis of a consequentialist principle:

"When we make decisions, the option we should choose is the one which maximizes expected value."[9] A consistent application of this principle, too, leads to a rejection of PB because the expected value of spending money on PB is simply not on a par with the expected value of using those same funds for other purposes—to alleviate poverty, for example.

At least three factors are relevant in making a decision according to a consequentialist view of expected value: the relative importance of the goods one must choose between; the number of people who will benefit; and the likelihood of the benefit. On each score, consistent consequentialists ought to choose alleviation of poverty ahead of PB. First, consider the significance of the goods involved. Given a choice between being deprived of the goods that procreative beneficence may deliver—such as greater intelligence—and being deprived of necessities for living—such as food, shelter, and basic medical care—virtually no one would choose to be without the basic necessities. The value of not sustaining life outweighs the value of greater intelligence. Therefore, developing and deploying procreative beneficence is not morally on par with helping to prevent suffering and death from lack of food, shelter, and basic medical care.

Second, if the benefits are equal, helping more people takes precedence over helping fewer people. Likewise, actual people take precedence over potential people (human embryos being, in the view of Savulescu and Kahane, potential people). Savulescu and Kahane endorse this principle: "As means of selection become safer and our ability to use them to select non-disease characteristics increases, we believe that PB will require most reproducers to select the most advantaged child *unless doing so is predicted to lead to a very significant loss of well-being to existing people*."[10] This is precisely the situation in which we find ourselves currently and for the foreseeable future. The financial resources used to benefit only one or two children through PB could instead be used to benefit more people living in poverty. The costs of IVF and PGD are high, averaging from $12,500 to $16,000 per cycle.[11] If, instead of spending this money to promote the well-being of one or two parents and the babies brought to live birth by IVF and PGD, the money were used to supply safe water, mosquito nets, and healthy food for people suffering in poverty, then the well-being of a greater number of people would be enhanced.

This conclusion might be avoided by appealing to the distinction between intentionally causing some effect and simply allowing the effect to occur. Although parents acting in accordance with PB may foresee that harm to those in poverty will be a side effect of their decision, their intention is not to harm people in poverty, but rather to benefit their child.

According to consequentialist doctrine, however, the distinction between intending and foreseeing harm is morally irrelevant. Savulescu holds, "A parent who intentionally inflicted deafness on his or her child, or failed to treat it, would be abusing the child. . . . There is no difference morally speaking between causing a harm and deliberately and avoidably allowing it to occur."[12] According to this view, there is therefore no moral difference between intentionally causing people in poverty to die by destroying their food or omitting to feed them,[13] which is the consequence of using $12,500 to $16,000 per cycle for IVF rather than for poverty relief.

This denial of the ethical difference between intending and objectively allowing a harmful effect causes problems for situating PB with respect to ethical and legal duties. Savulescu holds that PB is a moral duty, but not a legal one. Procreative autonomy, according to his view, is subject to moral, but not legal, proscription. But on what moral grounds, then, could we defend legislating against child abuse—for example, intentionally destroying a child's sight or hearing—but not criminalizing allowing a child to be deaf or blind? If intentionally doing and deliberately allowing are equivalent, then intentionally causing a child to be deaf and allowing her to be deaf should either both be legal or both be illegal. To decriminalize the act of blinding a child would be absurd, but to criminalize allowing a child to be born blind contradicts Savulescu's view of procreative autonomy.

Finally, by funding famine relief in lieu of procreative beneficence, money is more effectively spent in order to maximize expected utility. Resources spent on IVF and PDG usually do not bring about the desired benefit because more than 60% of the time IVF fails to lead to live birth. In contrast, supplying clean water, mosquito nets, and healthy food is virtually guaranteed to promote the well-being of those who need them. Furthermore, in a consequentialist framework, one cannot privilege benefit to oneself over benefit to others, so the fact that you seek to benefit your own child instead of famished strangers is ethically impermissible. Thus, if we have a duty to maximize expected well-being, then we have a duty not to use IVF and PDG for at least as long as conditions of famine and poverty exist anywhere in the world.

Rebecca Bennett criticizes PB from a different perspective. She argues that PB implicitly denies the fundamental dignity and equality of all human beings, including those with disabilities such as deafness or blindness.

> Any argument that a world without disabilities is not only preferable for many people, but is *morally* preferable, a morally better world, unavoidably rests on the assumption that a life with even moderate disabilities or impairments is a life with less moral value than other lives. We can understand that it is better for a particular person to have as good a quality of life as possible, but if we insist that a world without impaired people is morally preferable to a world containing impaired people, even though we admit that no one is harmed by being born in an impaired state, then we do so because we value the impaired less than the unimpaired. If the values placed on particular lives do not simply reflect many people's preferences but something of moral significance, then they must place a lower *moral* value on those lives impaired by a lower quality of life, whether this lower quality of life is as a result of disability, poverty, racial origins, aesthetic features, gender, etc.[14]

Advocates for PB insist that its underlying principle differs from eugenics because the goal is to produce the best child a couple could have, a private enterprise, rather than to produce the best society by selecting only the fittest humans to occupy it. Bennett challenges this assertion.

> As we have seen, the establishment of a moral obligation to bring to birth the best child we can is not built on the private interests of the prospective parents regarding what sort of child they wish to have, or on the individual interests of the child who will be created, as their welfare will not be affected by the decision about which embryo to

implant or which pregnancy to continue. What this obligation is built on is an idea of making the world a better place than it could otherwise have been, not in terms of any individual person's welfare, but in terms of creating the greatest total score for what is regarded as the goods of life. If a project is not interested in the welfare of particular people but in creating what those proposing this project believe is the best world possible, then this is exactly what eugenics is—promoting social and not personal goods.[15]

Bennett concludes by arguing that what matters morally is maximizing the welfare of actual people rather than choosing who is worthy of life among what she considers to be "potential" people, a decision based on the potential lives they might lead. If this is true, then as long as poverty or other financially amendable injustices exist in the world, PB is ethically impermissible.

In his article "The Illiberality of Perfectionist Enhancement," Teun Dekker suggests that liberalism and many eugenic enhancements are irreconcilable.[16] The liberal view, as described by Dekker, is that we may not impose our own conception of a good onto another person without that person's permission. This moral requirement binds governments as well as individuals, and it leads to liberal permissiveness in terms of legalizing drug use, same-sex marriage, physician-assisted suicide, and prostitution. However, insofar as procreative beneficence aims at enhancing any particular aptitude in a child—for instance, musical or athletic ability—such eugenics is illiberal because the parents force their conception of a good life—for instance, a life consisting of musical or athletic performance—onto the child without the child's consent.

Dekker provides an extreme example to make his case against what he calls "Perfectionist Enhancement." Imagine parents who believe the castrato opera to be the highest form of human expression, and so decide to genetically engineer their son to have no testicles in order that he might be able to hit high notes even as an adult. Imagine that the adult child deeply desires to marry and become a biological father. In this case, the parents have damaged the child's well-being and undermined his autonomy. Dekker's case against genetic enhancements echoes earlier thoughts articulated by C. S. Lewis, who wrote that by "means of selective breeding, [future generations] are, without their concurring voice, made to be what one generation, for its own reasons, may choose to prefer. From this point of view, what we call Man's power over Nature turns out to be a power exercised by some men over other men with Nature as its instrument."[17] Such power of one human being over another human being is an implicit denial of equal human dignity.

Dekker allows and indeed requires what he calls "natural primary goods enhancement," augmentations that enhance well-being in any path of life rather than well-being in one particular path of life chosen by the parents and imposed on the children. What exactly is the distinction between perfectionist enhancement and natural goods enhancement? Dekker explains:

> If natural primary goods are genetic traits that are useful for any plan of life, the inverse correlate might be termed perfectionist natural goods. These are traits that are only useful for certain plans of life and may very well be detrimental to many others. They might include musical ability and specific types of athletic prowess. All genetic traits that are useful for some plans of life but not for others are included in this category. Hence the distinction between natural primary goods enhancement and perfectionist enhancement is a very clear one; if we can imagine a plan of life for which the proposed enhancement is not useful, it is not a natural primary good.[18]

But is there in fact an authentic distinction between natural primary goods and perfectionist enhancement? Savulescu and Kahane express doubt: "What makes it harder to lead a good life in one circumstance may make it easier in another. The atopic tendency which leads to asthma in the developed world protects against worm infestations in the undeveloped world. Deafness would be a positive advantage in an environment of extremely loud and distracting noise."[19] Although characteristically quite useful, greater memory, impulse control, humor, and patience can also place a person at a disadvantage in certain circumstances.[20] Even intelligence and education, so beneficial in many situations, can put a person at a disadvantage in some contexts. Consider a highbrow professor making small talk with uncultivated relatives who communicate almost exclusively in pop-culture banalities and material fallacies. If the professor were less intelligent and educated, this familial social context would be comfortable and perhaps even invigorating or personally meaningful, but in fact, it is just the opposite. Natural goods enhancement turns out not to be different in kind from perfectionist enhancement. Both are illiberal. Both contradict human dignity, what is due each person.

Is it intrinsically evil to choose an existing child based on genetic endowment? Imagine parents who have their choice of available newborns at an orphanage. Would it be ethically wrong for them to choose one baby over others because they believe that the baby has a superior genetic endowment? I cannot see how it would be intrinsically evil. But note how this situation differs from the reality of PB. In an orphanage, parents neither choose among their own biological children nor consign the undesired children to death.

Imagine, however, that children conceived on even days had better genetic characteristics than children conceived on odd days. Would it be wrong to choose to make love on even days so as to maximize the chances of the child having a better genetic endowment? There seems to be reason to justify such a practice. Actual parents have duties to their children to help them have a good life. For this reason and others, parental neglect is seriously wrong. Parenthood is a morally serious enterprise, and in order to be a good parent, preparations must be made even prior to a child coming into existence to help the child have a good life. To fail to prepare properly for becoming parents is, once the child comes into existence, to neglect actual parental duties.

Properly understood, Savulescu's principle is acceptable, but he inconsistently applies it and draws wrong conclusions from it. If PB did not presuppose using abortion or using IVF and PGD, if IVF did not increase the likelihood of disability, if the fundamental principle giving rise to PB were consistently applied such that only a married couple could legitimately procreate, and if the vast sums of money used for PB for the possible benefit of one or two people were not desperately needed elsewhere to help many people, then, in my opinion, maximizing the genetic well-being of a child carried out by morally legitimate means would be acceptable and not contrary to upholding human dignity. However, without these qualifications, PB should be rejected.

In the future, reproductive technology may make PB a real possibility. Another future possibility is the gestation of a human being outside the uterus for the full term of pregnancy. To consider a slightly less extreme use of such technology, would it be ethically acceptable for a woman who no longer wanted to be pregnant to end her pregnancy not by abortion but by removal and gestation ex utero until full term of the child? Or to name another scenario, is it acceptable for a woman to begin a pregnancy by adopting and then gestating a human embryo? The next chapter focuses on these questions.

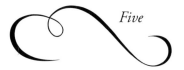

Five

Embryo Adoption and Artificial Wombs

Among those who accept the intrinsic dignity of every human being, disputes persist about whether the use of artificial wombs or the adoption of an embryo into a donor womb is permissible. In this chapter, I will offer a tentative assessment of the ethics of both embryo adoption (heterologous embryo transfer, or HET) and the use of an artificial uterus, taking into account currently articulated Catholic teaching. While embryo adoption is already a reality, a discussion of an artificial uterus may seem utterly speculative, akin to a moral evaluation of using a Star Trek transporter. Nevertheless, such a judgment must reckon with factual clinical developments. In 1973, fetal viability was considered to begin at around twenty-eight weeks of gestation, and neonates weighing less than 1,000 grams were allowed to die. But by the year 2000, premature infants of only eighteen weeks and 470 grams were reported to have survived.[1] Since then, efforts to lower the threshold of viability have continued (in particular at Temple University,[2] Cornell University,[3] and Juntendo University in Japan[4]). Given both the technological progress that can already save premature infants who have not been able to develop in utero during the typical gestational period and the teams of researchers who currently work to move the threshold of survivable premature birth back even further, the advent of artificial wombs seems less science fiction and more science future.

This chapter will examine the ethics of artificial wombs and embryo donation. In assessing the moral permissibility of the use of the artificial uterus and embryo adoption from the vantage point of the Catholic intellectual tradition, the official documents *Donum Vitae* (Instruction on Respect for Human Life), *Evangelium Vitae* (The Gospel of Life), and *Dignitas Personae* (The Dignity of the Person) are of special importance. These documents present the teachings of the Catholic Church on contemporary issues concerning the creation of human life, including in vitro fertilization (IVF), surrogate motherhood, and embryo experimentation.

It may seem to some that Catholic teaching already explicitly condemns embryo adoption. The case against embryo adoption rests on a passage from *Dignitas Personae:*

> The proposal that these embryos could be put at the disposal of infertile couples as a *treatment for infertility* is not ethically acceptable for the same reasons which make artificial heterologous procreation illicit as well as any form of surrogate motherhood; this practice would also lead to other problems of a medical, psychological and legal nature. It has also been proposed, solely in order to allow human beings to be born who are otherwise condemned to destruction, that there could be a form of *"prenatal adoption."* This proposal, praiseworthy with regard to the intention of respecting and defending human life, presents however various problems . . . .[5]

I believe that this passage presents a warning about the possible dangers of embryo adoption rather than a condemnation of the practice as intrinsically evil. *Dignitas Personae* says that embryo adoption is "problematic"; it does not say that it is "ethically impermissible" or "intrinsically evil." This document leaves the door open to consider ways in which these problematic elements might be mitigated. Despite the problems raised by embryo adoption, perhaps certain circumstances may justify the act as morally acceptable.

Although the official teaching office of the Catholic Church has never explicitly condemned artificial wombs or (according to my interpretation of *Dignitas Personae*) embryo adoption, it does provide principles that can be applied to both. Although these principles might initially seem to imply the moral impermissibility of both practices, I believe that nothing proposed by the Magisterium thus far necessarily leads to a comprehensive condemnation of either practice in all circumstances. Indeed, I believe fundamental principles of Catholic moral thought and accepted practice lead to the opposite conclusion.

In order to argue for this conclusion, several important arguments against artificial wombs and embryo adoption must be acknowledged: (1) the IVF objection; (2) the embryo transfer objection; (3) the integrative parenthood objection; (4) the marital unity objection; (5) the surrogate motherhood objection; and finally, (6) the wrongful experimentation objection. These objections suggest that the use of artificial wombs and the adoption of embryos are not morally acceptable. Although there is a great deal of plausibility to this view, after examining the teaching in greater detail, I believe this view to be incorrect.

In order to better assess how principles of Catholic teaching might apply to these cases, a terminological clarification is necessary because distinct—though sometimes related—matters should not be confused. By "complete ectogenesis," I mean the generation and development of a human being outside the womb continuously from the beginning of embryonic existence until the equivalent of forty weeks of gestation. By "partial ectogenesis," I mean the development of a human being outside the maternal womb during the typical gestational period, but not during the entire gestational period. An artificial womb could be used for either complete or partial ectogenesis. In other words, an artificial womb might be used to generate and sustain development of an embryo or fetus during the entire period of gestation or it might be used to sustain development after partial development within the maternal womb. By "embryo transfer" (ET) I mean the movement of an embryo that has never previously been implanted into an artificial womb or a maternal womb. By "heterologous embryo transfer" (HET) I mean the movement of an embryo into the womb of a woman who is not genetically related to the embryo. By "homologous embryo transfer" (HOT) I mean the movement of an embryo from a petri dish to a genetic mother's womb. By "fetal transfer" (FT) I mean the movement of a fetus from a maternal womb to either another maternal womb or to an artificial womb. Let us now consider some of the likely objections to artificial wombs or embryo adoption.

The In Vitro Fertilization Objection

The objections to IVF can be lodged against both embryo adoption and the use of an artificial uterus. As applied to embryo adoption, the IVF objection is that embryo adoption normalizes or regularizes IVF as a licit activity by demonstrating a tacit approval of IVF that is profiting, so to speak, from the wrongdoings of those who create life in the laboratory.

Embryo adoption does not in fact necessitate a tacit approval of IVF any more than normal adoption of a child conceived as a product of fornication, rape, or adultery indicates approval of these activities. Adoptions often involve some sort of prior wrongdoing on the part of the biological mother, father, or both, who brought about the conception of a child in circumstances in which they cannot properly provide for the child's well-being. Approval and promotion of adoption in such cases does not constitute the approval or promotion of the parents' wrongdoing itself but rather is often the most reasonable response to an imperfect situation brought about by human misconduct. The typical case of embryo adoption is, in other words, like the typical case of postnatal adoption.

The IVF objection to artificial wombs may be summarized as follows. The Catholic Church should oppose complete ectogenesis because it involves the use of cloning, parthenogenesis, or IVF in creating an embryo. From the perspective of *Donum Vitae,* these forms of creating human life are morally objectionable:

> Attempts or hypotheses for obtaining a human being without any connection with sexuality through "twin fission," cloning or parthenogenesis are to be considered contrary to the moral law, since they

are in opposition to the dignity both of human procreation and of the conjugal union. . . . Such fertilization (IVF) is in itself illicit and in opposition to the dignity of procreation and of the conjugal union, even when everything is done to avoid the death of the human embryo.[6]

Nevertheless, a condemnation of complete ectogenesis is not decisive for cases of partial ectogenesis because a woman seeking partial ectogenesis already has a human fetus within her. Partial ectogenesis does not involve fetal generation and development entirely outside the womb, but rather the continued development of an already generated human fetus transferred from a maternal womb to an artificial womb. In other words, it does follow from the fact that the Catholic Church opposes IVF, twin fission, cloning, or parthenogenesis that the Church would oppose complete ectogenesis, but it does not follow that it would necessarily oppose partial ectogenesis.

It could be argued that Pope John Paul II has already condemned partial ectogenesis. In his encyclical *Evangelium Vitae,* he wrote, "Among the most important of these rights, mention must be made of the right to life, an integral part of which is the right of the child to develop in the mother's womb from the moment of conception."[7] Does this passage condemn partial ectogenesis?

I am not convinced that an affirmative answer to this question is warranted. Nothing in this passage, indeed nothing of which I am aware in the writings of John Paul II, indicates that he had considered, let alone rejected, the use of artificial wombs as an alternative to abortion. Applying this single sentence, as if the pope had artificial wombs in mind, is not plausible. It is equally implausible to think that he would have condemned induction of labor just prior to the due date, a practice common in both Catholic and non-Catholic hospitals. Presumably, artificial wombs would be no more immoral than inducements of labor. Finally, the right of a child to develop in the womb from conception can be granted without also holding that this prima facie right holds in all conceivable circumstances and through all nine months of pregnancy. Artificial wombs would not violate this right so long as the health of both mother and child were not endangered.

The Embryo Transfer Objection

Another possible reason to condemn both the use of an artificial womb as well as embryo adoption is that both involve embryo transfer, a morally suspect practice.[8] Obviously, embryo adoption involves ET, for the embryo must be transferred from the cold-storage facility to the adoptive gestational mother's uterus. If embryo transfer is impermissible, then fetal transfer from a maternal womb to an artificial womb also seems impermissible. Because partial ectogenesis necessarily involves FT, it is wrong. It is important to note, however, that the condemnation of embryo transfer in *Donum Vitae* is always made in connection with IVF. The claim, therefore, could be that IVF and ET are objectionable as a combination, in which case ET alone might be found morally permissible.

In the case of embryo adoption (HET), it is not the same couple who create the new human being through IVF and then implant the developing human being in the womb. Although *Donum Vitae* condemns IVF, and although it excludes implantation into a surrogate mother, it does not explicitly condemn the reimplantation of an embryo created through IVF in the genetic mother's womb. It is counterintuitive to think that a couple who had already used IVF but repented of this wrongdoing has a further obligation not to implant any of the conceived human beings in the genetic mother's uterus. *Donum Vitae* asks that couples not create human beings via IVF, but does not explicitly declare ET per se illicit.

Indeed, there is reason to think that ET is not in itself illicit but rather is commendable in certain situations. Surgeons have, in very rare cases, removed an ectopic pregnancy from the site of implantation in the fallopian tube and reimplanted the developing human being in the uterus. Such cases of ET remove a grave health threat to the woman in question and also provide the only chance to preserve the life of the embryo itself. While most attempts at transplanting ectopic pregnancies unfortunately fail, there are a few recorded instances of successful births following the procedure.[9] Such efforts to save the developing human being in the case of ectopic pregnancy would seem to be morally permissible, so although HET may still be problematic, ET in itself is not objectionable. The alternative view, that ET is intrinsically evil, leads to the conclusion that one may not remove the human embryo from a location even if the embryo is doomed to die in that location and the mother's life is threatened, and even though moving the embryo would alleviate both problems. It is difficult to see how respect for both human embryonic and maternal life can justify such a conclusion.

If ET were unacceptable for any reason, then embryo adoption, too, would be impermissible because it necessarily involves ET as a means. However, simply because ET is ethically impermissible, it would not follow that fetal transfer (FT) is also problematic. After all, an emergency cesarean section of a premature baby in danger of dying is not morally problematic, and in some situations it may even be morally obligatory. Incubators now equate to primitive artificial wombs insofar as they are vital to help babies survive premature birth. As incubator technology advances, premature babies who die today will be viable tomorrow. So the use of artificial wombs, partial ectogenesis, or highly advanced incubators is not in principle prohibited by Catholic teaching.

The Integrative Parenthood Objection

Donum Vitae defends the importance of "integrative parenthood," and from this basis, one can also form objections to embryo adoption and partial ectogenesis.

> The child has the right to be conceived, carried in the womb, brought into the world and brought up within marriage: it is through the secure and recognized relationship to his own parents that the child can discover his own identity and achieve his own proper human development.[10]

Artificial insemination using gametes from someone outside the marriage is impermissible for the same reason:

> Heterologous artificial fertilization violates the rights of the child; it deprives him of his filial relationship with his parental origins and can hinder the maturing of his personal identity. Furthermore, it

offends the common vocation of the spouses who are called to fatherhood and motherhood: it objectively deprives conjugal fruitfulness
of its unity and integrity; it brings about and manifests a rupture between genetic parenthood, gestational parenthood and responsibility
for upbringing.[11]

Embryo adoption is therefore understood to constitute an injustice done
to the child by causing a rupture between genetic and gestational motherhood. In the words of Catherine Althaus, a woman choosing embryo
adoption "seeks to separate genetic motherhood from gestational motherhood and deny the embryo the dignity appropriate to its development
and human existence."[12] At first glance, these considerations also seem to
exclude any use of artificial wombs as undermining gestational parenthood, which is important in securing the well-being of the child. We
could call this the integrative parenthood objection to ectogenesis. In
other words, integrative parenthood involves not separating genetic parenthood from gestational parenthood, and entails the responsibility for
raising and rearing the child—what might be called social parenthood.
Thus, it is contrary to the union of husband and wife to have a child via
embryo adoption and also contrary to the child's right to *integrative parenthood* to practice embryo adoption or the use of an artificial womb
because it deprives the developing human being of a unified genetic, gestational, and social parenthood.

Although on first consideration the integrative parenthood objection
would seem to exclude both embryo adoption and the use of an artificial
uterus, I believe that the interpretation of integrative parenthood offered
by critics is too strong to accord with other accepted practices. If this
right to be conceived, gestated, and reared within marriage were understood to mean that every child once conceived must be brought up within
the marriage in which he or she was conceived, it would follow that all
women who find themselves pregnant outside of marriage (even by rape)
must marry the father. Although in many cases of extramarital pregnancy,
a marriage of father and mother constitutes the best response to the situation, marriage following pregnancy is not always advisable, let alone a
moral duty. In some cases of extramarital pregnancy, marriage is not only
gravely imprudent but indeed would not be permissible or even possible,

such as when a pregnancy occurs as the result of incest or when a prior valid marriage exists for one or both of the parties in question.

Moreover, if the right to integrative parenthood is understood as the right for every existing child to be nurtured in his or her mother's womb until full-term birth and then to be reared by the married biological parents, it would follow that every birth mother placing a child for adoption and every couple accepting an adopted child would be doing something wrong. The *Instruction* specifically notes, however, that far from being an evil choice, adoption is an important service to life: "Physical sterility in fact can be for spouses the occasion for other important services to the life of the human person, for example, adoption, various forms of educational work, and assistance to other families and to poor or handicapped children."[13] Birth mothers who generously and bravely place their child in another family through adoption in consideration of the child's best interest perform a loving and heroic act, and those who adopt children likewise perform a generous act.

Donum Vitae is therefore best understood as proposing that one should not *cause a human being to come into existence* unless one can nurture the child in the womb prior to birth and properly care for the child after birth. A child's right to integrative parenthood involves the marriage of the child's mother and father, the conception of the child by husband and wife in the act of marriage, the nurturing of the child within the maternal womb, and then the raising of the child by his or her biological parents.

Once conception has taken place, however, it is in certain circumstances permissible, and even praiseworthy, to allow the child to be adopted if this option is prudentially judged to be in the best interest of the individual child. Although it would be wrong to conceive a child solely in order to place him or her for adoption, the Catholic Church's ongoing support of adoption makes it clear that it is not always wrong, and in many cases it is indeed commendable, to turn to adoption following the conception of a child. It does not seem to be morally relevant whether the adoption takes place at forty weeks (after full gestation), at twenty-five weeks (as a result of premature birth), by use of an artificial womb at seven weeks, or by way of embryo adoption at seven days, so long as the well-being of the mother and the child is not endangered. The couple who make the embryo adoption do not seek to separate genetic motherhood from gestational motherhood. The separation was already chosen, previously forced upon the child, when the biological parents abandoned the embryo. Embryo adoption does not deny the embryo the dignity appropriate to its development and human existence but, given our current technology, rather secures this dignity in the only way possible at such an early stage of human development. The right of a child to integrative parenthood may apply prior to conception, but clearly this right is disposed to exceptions that will secure for the already existing child more fundamental rights, such as the right to life itself.

The Marital Unity Objection

This objection to embryo adoption focuses on the marital unity of the husband and wife's relationship, at least as potential mother and father to a child. *Donum Vitae* notes: "The fidelity of spouses in the unity of marriage involves reciprocal respect of their right to become a father and a mother only through each other."[14] From this and other passages, some argue that it is against the marital unity of spouses for a married woman to become pregnant with a child that is not the fruit of her marriage. Nicholas Tonti-Filippini, for example, argues that embryo adoption is excluded in this case because the woman becomes pregnant, and thus a mother, through someone other than her husband.[15]

This view is in some tension with aspects of Catholic revelation, indeed its most central proclamation that God became a human being. If it were an exceptionless norm that a woman may become pregnant only by her husband, the "fiat" of Mary becomes morally problematic. Aquinas holds that the Virgin Mary was truly married to Joseph.[16] Though this marriage was never consummated sexually, Mary and Joseph did share a true marriage bond. According to Aquinas's view, at the time of the Annunciation Mary was already married to Joseph, not merely engaged, and consented to become pregnant with a child that was not the fruit of her marriage to Joseph. There is some division among the Fathers of the Church as to whether Mary was guilty of any personal sin whatsoever. A few Greek Fathers assert that she did sin personally, but the Western tradition of Augustine, Aquinas, the Council of Trent, and Pius XII holds that she was free from not only original sin (via the Immaculate Conception) but also personal sin. There is in any case universal agreement among Christian believers that in her consent to become the mother of God, Mary did not sin. Of course, unlike cases of heterologous embryo adoption Jesus and Mary were genetically related. But this consideration is irrelevant to the marital unity objection if a woman becomes pregnant by a man other than her husband. One might argue that Mary was the spouse of the Holy Spirit and not of Joseph at the time of the Annunciation. This view, however, would present the problem that by marrying Joseph, Mary either had two husbands or divorced the Holy Spirit. A related point is made by John Stanmeyer, who focuses on the real and adoptive fatherhood of Joseph.[17] Obviously, the Annunciation and the Holy Family are special cases, but we can also consider other, less singular cases.

One such example, which unlike the Annunciation is neither singular nor divine, is a married woman who is raped during her fertile period. Such a woman might have good reason to believe that she may have conceived a child, but that the embryo might not have yet implanted in her womb. If it is an exceptionless moral norm that one should become impregnated (in the sense of having an embryo implant) only by one's spouse, then this woman would be under a moral obligation to use an abortifacient drug to prevent the implantation of the newly conceived embryo. Obviously, there is no duty to use an abortifacient; indeed, there is a duty not to use an abortifacient. Sarah-Vaughan Brakman argues this point, citing that the prohibition of post-rape therapy that would prevent implantation undercuts Pacholczyk's argument that even the genetic parents of frozen embryos should not consent to implantation.[18] The two cases are of course not entirely comparable: a rape lacks voluntary consent, but embryo adoption involves informed consent.

In addition, embryo adoption does respect the right of spouses to become parents only through one another. Parenthood can be distinguished into various aspects, as noted: genetic, gestational, and social. In the case of embryo adoption, the parents do not become genetic parents through anyone other than each other, which is precisely the situation that *Donum Vitae* addresses. With respect to postbirth adoption, however, the social parents take on the responsibility for a child whose existence they did not initiate but whose needs they have promised to meet. The adoptive mother does not become a biological mother through someone other than her husband, and the husband does not become a biological father through someone other than his wife. Together, they both become parents—adoptive parents—by means of another couple. Similarly, in embryo adoption, the social father and gestational-social mother agree to take on responsibility for the well-being of the human embryo. A woman does not become a biological mother through embryo adoption, so she does not undermine the goods of marital unity any more than do parents who adopt after birth. Adoptive parents do not violate a prohibition on becoming genetic parents through another who is not their spouse be-cause the adoptive parents never become the genetic parents of the child they adopt. They become parents of another couple's genetic child.

Another version of the marital unity objection holds that gestation is included as an aspect of the conjugal act, the exercise of which should be reserved exclusively to the husband and wife.[19] According to this view, for example, Pacholczyk argues that procreation includes pregnancy, so those who choose HET separate the procreative act from the unitive act of sex-ual intercourse much as do those who practice IVF.[20]

E. Christian Brugger has indicated several challenges to the argument that pregnancy is part of procreation. First, it is in tension with the idea that a new human being comes into existence when fertilization is com-plete. When there is a new human being, procreation has already taken place. If procreation—the creation of a new human being—is considered to last throughout gestation, then abortion would not really kill an inno-cent human being.[21] Second, gestation is a period of development of the human child, which implies that the human being is already in existence, and hence that procreation has been completed.[22] Third, why should "procreation" in the sense meant by Pacholczyk, who understands it really as an aspect of human development, be said to end at birth if the process of human development continues during infancy and beyond? Unless human development ended at birth, this would deem not only embryo adoption but also traditional adoption immoral.[23] Finally, there are no biological, philosophical, or theological grounds for positing that the en-tire period of gestation constitutes an ongoing process of procreation.[24]

It is more difficult still to see how artificial wombs would undermine marital unity if used after the onset of normal pregnancy. If a woman finds herself pregnant, but in the course of pregnancy it is medically determined that the pregnancy is failing, then advanced incubation systems may serve—just as our less advanced intensive care units for premature infants currently serve—to preserve the fragile human life that has begun. Creating human life outside the womb and continuing to gestate that life outside the womb would be a different matter, for it would necessarily involve using IVF or other immoral techniques of creating human life. This case is distinct from that of premature infants whose lives cannot in practice be sustained with the current technology but who theoretically could be saved by highly advanced neonatal care units (artificial wombs). Thus, I would argue that it is morally wrong to create human life outside the womb and gestate this life in an artificial uterus, but it is morally permissible (indeed morally good) to save endangered human life via an artificial uterus in cases where a natural pregnancy is failing.

The more difficult question, namely, whether artificial wombs should be used to gestate currently frozen human embryos (rather than just to rescue failing pregnancies in progress), is an important question, but it is one that I shall not attempt to answer in this chapter. I would expect that the same objections that are raised to HET would be raised to the use of artificial wombs in such cases, but fully considering these objections (which very well may be successful against the use of artificial wombs but not against HET to save frozen embryos) falls outside the scope of this inquiry. Of particular concern is the possibility of abuse of the embryo, for a human being abandoned by his or her biological parents and without a gestational mother would potentially be prey to the very worst kinds of abuse: for example, the harvesting of organs for transplantation and medical experimentation. On the other hand, were I to be a frozen embryo, I would (if I could choose) prefer to be implanted in an artificial uterus, brought to maturity for nine months, and then be adopted, rather than to remain frozen or, worse, be killed or allowed to die. These concerns, both pro and con, cannot however be adequately addressed as part of the question at hand. I turn now to another objection to both artificial wombs and embryo adoption.

The Surrogate Mother Objection

Taking a different approach to these issues, one might argue that if surrogate motherhood is wrong, then both embryo adoption and the use of an artificial uterus must also be wrong. *Donum Vitae* clearly indicates that surrogate motherhood is morally impermissible:

> Surrogate motherhood represents an objective failure to meet the obligations of maternal love, of conjugal fidelity and of responsible motherhood; it offends the dignity and the right of the child to be conceived, carried in the womb, brought into the world and brought up by his own parents; it sets up, to the detriment of families, a division between the physical, psychological and moral elements which constitute those families.[25]

If surrogate motherhood is wrong, and if embryo adoption and partial ectogenesis are forms of surrogate motherhood and indeed artificial motherhood, then ectogenesis is also wrong. This may be called the surrogate motherhood objection to embryo adoption and partial ectogenesis.

In considering this objection, it is important to specify how *Donum Vitae* defines surrogate motherhood. A surrogate mother is defined as:

> (a) the woman who carries in pregnancy an embryo implanted in her uterus and who is genetically a stranger to the embryo because it has been obtained through the union of the gametes of "donors." She carries the pregnancy with a pledge to surrender the baby once it is born to the party who commissioned or made the agreement for the pregnancy.
> (b) the woman who carries in pregnancy an embryo to whose procreation she has contributed the donation of her own ovum, fertilized through insemination with the sperm of a man other than her husband. She carries the pregnancy with a pledge to surrender the child once it is born to the party who commissioned or made the agreement for the pregnancy.[26]

Neither definition includes embryo adoption or partial ectogenesis as a form of surrogate motherhood. In the case of embryo adoption, the gestational mother does not make a pledge to surrender the child once it is born (an element in both definitions of surrogacy in *Donum Vitae*); rather, she intends to rear the child as the social mother.[27] Indeed, embryo adoption can be viewed as approximating the ideal of integrative parenthood. In embryo adoption, the same woman is the gestational and social mother, whereas in a typical adoption, the woman who rears the child did not gestate the baby.

The definitions of surrogacy offered in *Donum Vitae* would exclude the use of an artificial uterus in some circumstances. Both definitions speak of the transfer of an embryo, but partial ectogenesis does not necessarily involve embryo transfer (ET) as I have defined it (the movement of an embryo that has never previously been implanted into an artificial womb or a maternal womb) because it can and most likely involves moving the human fetus from a maternal womb to an artificial womb. Furthermore, both definitions of surrogate motherhood involve pledges by the surrogate mother to surrender the baby once it is born to the party who commissioned or made the agreement for the pregnancy. Obviously, an artificial womb cannot pledge or agree to anything, nor does partial ectogenesis always necessarily involve giving the baby to those who initiated creation of the baby. Indeed, in typical cases, the woman who otherwise would have chosen abortion does not want to or cannot rear the baby. Furthermore, surrogate motherhood, according to the definitions given in *Donum Vitae,* necessarily involves IVF; as was mentioned earlier, partial ectogenesis does not. Hence, the impermissibility of surrogate motherhood as understood in *Donum Vitae* does not entail the impermissibility of using highly advanced incubators in lieu of abortion.

The Wrongful Experimentation Objection

Even if all the previous objections can be overcome, embryo adoption and partial ectogenesis—at least before the fetus is well developed—would seem to involve wrongful experimentation. Pope John Paul II writes in *Evangelium Vitae:*

> This [negative] evaluation of the morality of abortion is to be applied also to the recent forms of intervention on human embryos which, although carried out for purposes legitimate in themselves, inevitably involve the killing of those embryos. This is the case with experimentation on embryos, which is becoming increasingly widespread in the field of biomedical research and is legally permitted in some countries. Although one must uphold as licit procedures carried out on the human embryo which respect the life and integrity of the embryo and do not involve disproportionate risks for it, but rather are directed to its healing, the improvement of its condition of health, or its individual survival, it must nonetheless be stated that the use of human embryos or fetuses as an object of experimentation constitutes a crime against their dignity as human beings who have a right to the same respect owed to a child once born, just as to every person.[28]

If experimentation on human beings before birth is licit only if directed to the healing, the improvement of its condition or health, or the individual survival of the embryo or fetus, then to attempt partial ectogenesis would be wrong. Use of artificial wombs in lieu of abortion would subject the human fetus to risks not for the sake of the fetus's own welfare, but for the sake of the mother being free from pregnancy. Even if techniques of partial ectogenesis are eventually made routine, all early attempts at partial ectogenesis would be wrongful experimentation.

It would indeed be a case of wrongful experimentation to create a human embryo for the sake of implantation in a gestational mother's uterus for the purpose of adoption. This would create an embryo only to needlessly subject it to risks. However, in the situation of embryo adoption in which the human embryo has already been brought into existence and is left over from IVF treatments, embryo adoption is currently the only possible means of survival for the embryo and so is not contrary to the interests of the embryo. Indeed, embryo adoption is precisely the only currently available means to ensure the "individual survival" of the embryo, to use the language of *Evangelium Vitae,* and so does not constitute forbidden experimentation on the embryo.

As others have pointed out with respect to an artificial uterus, ecto-genesis could be developed naturally as an extension of saving premature babies. Experimental procedures undertaken to save the life of premature babies are acceptable given the principles suggested by John Paul II be-cause they would be directed towards the individual survival of the pre-mature babies in question. As these techniques are improved by means of this acceptable experimentation, eventually partial ectogenesis may occur very early in pregnancy as a common procedure that does not expose its human subjects to any disproportionate risks. Indeed, one can imagine ectogenesis becoming *less risky* than normal gestation because an artificial womb would not, presumably, be subject to accidents such as car crashes, slips and falls, or criminal assault, as might a womb inside of a woman. In other words, accepting that experimentation should only be undertaken for the good of the one experimented upon still leaves room for the legiti-mate development of artificial wombs if these artificial wombs are devel-oped in the process of trying to save premature infants who would other-wise die. For the many couples who can conceive a child but have difficulty bringing a pregnancy to full term, highly advanced incubators would help to remedy a deficiency present in nature and so would be ar-tificial in the best sense of the term.

In my opinion, the IVF objection, the embryo transfer objection, the integrative parenthood objection, the surrogate motherhood objection, and finally, the wrongful experimentation objection all fail to show the impermissibility of either embryo adoption for embryos already in exis-tence or the use of artificial wombs in lieu of abortion.

My remarks thus far have sought to remove very reasonable, but what I believe are ultimately mistaken, objections to embryo adoption and partial ectogenesis based on extrapolations from magisterial Catholic teaching. But what would be the positive case for embryo adoption and partial ectogenesis? Although they may not be wrong in light of recent Catholic teaching on bioethical questions, what reason do we have to be-lieve they are permissible courses of action?

The most obvious answer is that both practices could save innocent human life. Although there is no exact data on the matter, there are more than 400,000 frozen human embryos in the United States. The only cur-rently available chance they have to grow to human maturity is through embryo adoption. Indeed, most such embryos will not remain permanently frozen and will die when removed from deep freeze. The general duty of promoting and protecting life suggests the value of embryo adoption.

Likewise, the limited use of artificial wombs could save many human lives. Each year, there are approximately 43 million abortions worldwide and between 1.2 and 1.6 million in the United States alone. If only a small percentage of abortions were eliminated by using artificial wombs, this would be a great service to the human community. Like orphanages, which have long been sponsored by the Church, support of highly advanced incubators would help preserve the well-being of innocent human persons who otherwise would be lost.

Both embryo adoption and partial ectogenesis could also be great services to many women. Embryo adoption allows infertile couples the chance to become parents and infertile women to have the experience of gestational parenthood. Most couples who adopt prefer, I would say reasonably, to adopt babies rather than older children so as to form a bond with the child from the very beginning of life outside the womb. For similar reasons, many couples seeking to adopt would like to begin fostering that bond with the new member of the family even earlier, in the first months of life in utero.

Likewise, advanced incubators (artificial wombs) would help many married couples who repeatedly lose pregnancies prior to natural viability due to maternal health problems or various kinds of maternal-fetal incompatibility or pathology. Those who allege that the Church's teaching on abortion arises from an explicit or implicit desire to subjugate women by tying them down to pregnancy do not realize that the teaching arises from an affirmation of the equality and dignity of every single human being. It is precisely care and concern for the well-being of all human beings that leads to a condemnation of abortion; this same care and concern for all people leads to the approval of highly advanced incubators in lieu of abortion. The foreseen effects of forgoing abortion in cases of crisis pregnancy are characteristically much more difficult for the women involved than for the men. Often, not choosing abortion calls those involved to heroic generosity. Because the Church is committed to helping all people develop morally and in their compassion for others, the Church as an institution already works to lessen the difficulties involved in such crisis pregnancy situations by offering homes for mothers in need, providing child care, and making other material and spiritual support available. Approval of partial ectogenesis would be an extension of these efforts to ease the burdens placed uniquely on pregnant women.

Consider this thought experiment: What if instead of considering the use of highly advanced incubators in lieu of abortion, we had discovered an injection that sped up the time of gestation? Rather than nine months of pregnancy, a woman who received this injection would be able to give birth to a full-term, perfectly healthy baby nine minutes later. Suppose the injection was only as risky for mothers and their babies as normal childbirth, so that it posed no greater risk than the alternative of continuing pregnancy at the normal rate. Would use of such injections be condemned as intrinsically evil by the Church?

I think the answer would be no. Although the injections would hardly be natural, they are no more contrary to nature than pain medication to ease the agony of labor. Rather than enduring morning sickness, interruption of educational or work schedules, and other hardships associated with nine months of pregnancy, women would be able to forgo these difficulties, if they chose, giving due consideration for all the goods involved, especially the well-being of the child in question. Women who might otherwise choose abortion rather than adoption due to the long months of bonding with the child that would make placing the child for adoption extremely difficult would be able to place their babies with another family before extensive bonding developed. Those who would choose abortion out of shame could speed up the gestation and deliver before anyone found out. Rape victims would not have to be reminded for nine months of their sexual assault. In other words, women would be helped; children would be preserved. These considerations apply equally well to the use of artificial wombs as an alternative to abortion. Whether such an injection would be permissible in typical situations of pregnancy is another question. Whether such an injection would also be permissible to "speed up" other stages of human life such as infancy or childhood is yet another question. For both parents and children, there are goods intrinsic to the practices of bearing or raising children in a normal way.

Needless to say, there are also serious questions and perhaps insurmountable obstacles to developing such an injection in a morally permissible way. However, there are very few—indeed extremely few—classes of actions (e.g., murder, adultery, perjury, apostasy) that are deemed by the Church to be intrinsically evil, and it is hard to see why an injection speeding pregnancy would fall into the category of deeds never to be done no matter what the consequences. Like placing a newborn or an older child for adoption, it would not, in my opinion, be intrinsically evil even though it should not be taken lightly.

The phrases "embryo adoption" and "artificial wombs" conjure images of Huxley's *Brave New World* or scenes from *Star Wars: Attack of the Clones*. A dehumanized family dehumanizes civilization. The case of embryo adoption, however, makes the best of an already imperfect situation. In an ideal world, all children would be created as the fruit of the love between a husband and wife. In reality, and as we have discussed, sometimes children are conceived in ways that do not do justice to their fundamental needs and dignity as flourishing or attributed. Obviously, the immoral circumstances of these types of conception do not change the intrinsic dignity and worth of the one who is conceived. When conception takes place in such circumstances, it is sometimes best for those involved that the child be placed for adoption. It makes no important moral difference whether this adoption takes place earlier or later in the child's life, though from the perspective of the child, it would seem that the earlier the adoption takes place, the better. If the adoption can take place at the very beginning of life, if the social mother can also become the gestational mother, then so much the better for that child.

Likewise, the artificial uterus is no more ominous than highly advanced versions of the neonatal intensive care units widely used today to save the lives of thousands of premature infants. Like any technology, it could possibly be abused, but abuse does not undermine legitimate use. Each year in the United States, nearly half a million births—more than ten percent—take place at or before thirty-six weeks. Although at present saving these children is very expensive and many of them become seriously disabled, we can hope that both of these drawbacks might be eliminated in the future. In other words, we have primitive artificial wombs and stone-age partial ectogenesis right now—and they are accepted by everyone. The use of technologically advanced incubators in lieu of abortion is therefore also morally acceptable, especially when the other likely alternative ends with a dead child and a wounded woman. In sum, I believe that both embryo adoption and the use of an artificial womb are morally permissible in some circumstances as manifestations of our care for the vulnerable, especially at the beginning of life.

Unfortunately, not only choice but also accidents of nature can endanger the life of a human being. In an ectopic pregnancy, an embryo lodges outside the uterus and continues development, threatening the lives of both the mother and the developing embryo. The ethics of managing such situations remains a vexing problem for ethicists committed to the equal dignity of all human beings. The next chapter examines the ethics of ectopic pregnancy.

Six

The Ethics of Ectopic Pregnancy

If all human beings, including those in utero, deserve to be respected and treated with the human dignity accorded to every person, how then should cases of ectopic pregnancy be treated? Among those who accept that all human beings deserve equal human rights, there remains a lively debate about how to handle such cases. Extrauterine or ectopic pregnancies occur outside the uterus; the vast majority of these are found in the fallopian tube. As the pregnancy continues, the fallopian tube may burst and cause hemorrhaging which can lead to maternal death. It is estimated that in the United States alone, ectopic pregnancy is the number one cause of maternal fatality in the first trimester of pregnancy and results in the death of about forty to fifty women each year.[1]

In some cases of ectopic pregnancy, the embryo has already died, but the trophoblast—the forerunner to the placenta—continues to bore into the fallopian tube. In cases in which the embryo has died but the placenta continues to build—so-called "persistent ectopic pregnancy"—any medically indicated treatment to save the mother is morally permissible because the child is no longer alive. If we define the term as Pope John Paul II did, "direct" abortion—that is, abortion willed as an end or as a means—is always wrong because it is the deliberate (i.e., intentional) killing of an innocent human being.[2] Of course, once the human embryo or human fetus has died, direct abortion is no longer at issue, so any safe means of removing the embryonic remains and other products of conception from the formerly expectant mother is morally acceptable.

How should ectopic pregnancies in which the human embryo is still alive be treated? How should health care providers and hospitals committed to the basic equal dignity of all human beings respond to this medical emergency?

In current medical practice, the following methods are used to treat tubal pregnancy:

(1) expectant management
(2) removal of the tube with the embryo inside it (salpingectomy)
(3) removal of the embryo alone while leaving the tube intact (salpingostomy)
(4) administration of methotrexate

In this chapter, I will discuss these procedures in order to determine which of these treatments may be licitly practiced by those who affirm that every single human being should be protected by law and welcomed into life.

Expectant Management

In expectant management, nature is allowed to take its course in hope that the situation will resolve itself. In some 40% to 64% of these cases, a tubal pregnancy spontaneously aborts, and the threat to the mother's life is removed without the physician having to resort to surgical or chemical intervention.[3] With expectant management, the pregnant woman is carefully monitored by means of serial hormone levels and ultrasounds. If the embryo grows and the mother's hormone levels continue to rise, then some intervention is medically indicated, and expectant management is a morally permissible way to treat tubal pregnancy in many cases. Where expectant management is no longer medically indicated, other treatment options should be used.

Salpingectomy: Removal of the Tube with the Embryo Inside

This proposal is widely accepted as an application of the principle of double effect. Double-effect reasoning applies to this case as follows.

(1) Considered by itself and independently of its effects, the action of removing the damaged fallopian tube is not evil. As in the case of removing a cancerous uterus, the fallopian tube has become pathological and a threat to the health of the woman. It is a good action to alleviate pathology, even if it means excising once-healthy organs.
(2) The evil of the embryo's death is not a means to the good but rather a side effect of the morally legitimate goal of stopping or preventing maternal bleeding.
(3) The evil of embryonic death is not intended as an end. The removal of the tube is not a pretext for bringing about the death of the embryo.
(4) Finally, there is a proportionate reason for allowing the evil effect because without the surgical intervention, the mother may die, and the embryo will die even without the intervention.

These two procedures—expectant management and removal of the fallopian tube (or section of the fallopian tube) with the embryo inside it—have found nearly universal acceptance by those committed to the basic equality of all human beings from conception to natural death. Unfortunately, removal of the fallopian tube diminishes the potential fertility of the woman, and in cases where problems already exist with the other tube, she may be rendered sterile.

Salpingostomy: Removal of the Embryo While Leaving the Tube Intact

The medical advantage of removing only the embryo is that the fallopian tube remains intact, thus able to facilitate future pregnancies. Because the life of the embryo is almost certain to be lost, many ethicists reason that it makes sense to preserve what can still be preserved—namely the woman's capacity for fertility. This can be done by salpingostomy. Ethicists are divided about whether this procedure constitutes direct abortion.[4] At least three arguments support the view that removal of the embryo alone is intrinsically evil, yet each of those three arguments fails to withstand critical scrutiny.

A first objection to salpingostomy is that removing the embryo alone, rather than the pathological tube with the embryo in it, is direct abortion because it is certainly fatal for the embryo. These procedures bring about death for the embryo with certainty, so they must be intentionally or directly killing the embryo. However, most ethicists also agree that if a woman discovers she has uterine cancer, she may have the uterus removed even if she is pregnant with a baby that is not yet viable.[5] In other words, she may have the cancerous uterus removed even if it is certain that the pre-viable unborn child will die. Removal of the uterus is not intentionally killing the unborn, despite the certain side effect of fetal death. So the fact that a given medical procedure brings about fetal death with certainty does not mean that it is intentional or direct abortion. Similarly, the removal of the pathological tube along with the human embryo (salpingectomy) also causes certain embryonic death, so the certainty of death by no means indicates that the procedure is intentional abortion.

Second, it is sometimes argued that removal of the human embryo from the tube simply is the very same thing as killing the embryo, just as the act of cutting off someone's head simply is killing the person. But what if the human embryo could be successfully removed and implanted in the uterus? Some claim that this procedure has already taken place successfully. In the *American Journal of Obstetrics and Gynecology,* L. Shettles reports:

> In Gifford Memorial Hospital, Randolph, Vermont, in 1980, a 27-year-old patient with unaccountable infertility and regular 28-day cycles had intercourse around the middle of the month. Approximately 4 weeks later severe pain developed in the region of the left fallopian tube. . . . Exploration while the patient was under regional anesthesia revealed a single corpus luteum in the left ovary, some uterine congestion, and on the direct palpation of the left tube a

small 4 to 5 mm mass. With careful incision into the tubal lumen, an intact embryonic sac was enucleated, still completely covered with chorionic villi. . . . It was immediately placed in an oxygenated saline solution warmed to body temperature. A segment of infusion tubing was cut, one end slanting and the other attachable to a glass Preto syringe with a large rubber bulb enabling one to aspirate or express as desired. With gentle suction the slanted end of the tubing was passed into the myometrium in the upper, anterior aspect of the uterus until discernible decidual tissue was observed. With the tubing in situ, the embryonic sac was taken up into the glass syringe, which was then attached to the tubing and expressed in utero. Tamponade of the puncture side with a very wa[r]m pad controlled any bleeding. The tube was then repaired and the abdomen closed. The pregnancy test remained positive. After a normal postoperative and prenatal course, a normal infant was delivered at term.[6]

If this report and another much older one like it are accurate,[7] salpingostomy does not necessarily involve the death of the embryo. In other words, removing the embryo from the fallopian tube in itself is not simply the same thing as intentionally killing the embryo. Although there is not yet an established protocol for this transfer, one can hope that advances in microsurgery and early detection of tubal pregnancy will make possible both a preservation of the embryonic human being and the reproductive capability of the fallopian tube.

Indeed, the removal of the embryo from its pathological site of implantation by surgical removal of the embryo alone (salpingostomy) is implicitly recognized as a morally good or indifferent action, considered by itself and independently of its effects (the first condition of double effect) even by those who condemn these procedures. A number of respected ethicists vigorously oppose removing the embryo alone, including William E. May,[8] Eugene F. Diamond,[9] and Kelly Bowring,[10] but they nevertheless also endorse efforts at embryo transplantation from the fallopian tube to the uterus. Such transplantation, however, necessarily involves detaching the embryo from its location in the fallopian tube—which, if it were intrinsically evil (not merely from its effects) would therefore never be permissible to perform, regardless of the consequences. At least implicitly, these authors do not hold that detachment of the embryo from its pathological location is in itself intrinsically evil, or they should—to be consistent—condemn as intrinsically evil any effort to transplant a tubal pregnancy into the uterus.

One may object that it is immoral to remove the embryo from its pathological implantation site if one has no safe haven for the embryo, such as the uterus. To use a different example, it would not be wrong to take someone off a raft in order to put that person into a lifeboat, but it would be wrong to knock someone off a raft if there were no place to put him, even if the person were certain to die on the raft. According to this argument, because there is no feasible transplantation technique for ectopic pregnancy, the removal of the embryo is morally wrong. If there were such a technique, it would not be wrong to remove the embryo while leaving the tube intact.

However, if some further condition may accurately render an act moral and no longer evil, then it was not an intrinsically evil act. If something is intrinsically evil—as opposed to circumstantially evil—then no further circumstance can render that act good. This is the case with our example, which includes the further circumstance that the embryo can be removed to another place of safety. In other words, the response itself implicitly indicates that removing a human embryo from its point of pathological location is not intrinsically evil, just as removing someone from a raft is not intrinsically evil. Both may be circumstantially evil, but one must take into account the additional circumstances that disprove the act as intrinsically evil.

Some argue that removal of the embryo without the tube is illicit because it involves a physical manipulation of the body of the embryo that is not of benefit to the embryo, unlike removal of the tube along with the embryo, in which the maternal fallopian tube is the object of the intervention. In the words of May, in "the hysterectomy (and, similarly, the salpingectomy in handling a tubal pregnancy), the medical intervention is performed on the *mother*, whereas in the 'removals' of the unborn child by . . . . salpingostomy . . . the interventions are performed on the *unborn child*."[11]

The removal of the embryo from the fallopian tube does not, however, constitute an attack on the body of the human embryo, for it can be performed—although it is usually not—in such a way that the embryo's physical integrity is not undermined. Removal of the embryo from the pathological location of implantation could be effective such that the tubal maternal tissue that has been damaged is removed—leaving the embryo's bodily integrity intact.[12] Indeed, if transplantation is facilitated, the removal would constitute a therapeutic intervention for both the mother and the human embryo.

Even if the surgery were performed on the body of the human embryo, thus harming the human embryo's body, that would not in itself mean that the surgery was a direct or intentional abortion/killing. In reasoning about self-defense, Thomas Aquinas famously argued that the act of self-defense is morally permissible even though performed against the body of the attacker and even though death results from the defensive force used.[13] Obviously, the human embryo is not an "attacker" in the formal sense, but Aquinas's point remains that the use of lethal force against another's body does not in itself necessarily constitute intentional killing.

My point here is not to argue that the human embryo can be killed because the killing is justified as an act of self-defense. My point is that acting directly on someone's body does not, in itself, mean that all the effects of doing so are intended. In the case of a just war, a tactical bomber may drop a bomb that both intentionally destroys a legitimate military target and as a side effect impinges upon and kills innocent civilians. Such a bombing may be justified for a proportionate reason.[14] Conversely, there are some intentional killings in which no action is taken upon the body of the victim. For example, parents who intentionally omit to feed their baby in order to kill the infant intentionally kill but do not act upon the body of the baby. They deliberately omit an action that they could have and should have performed as a means to secure the death of an innocent person. In such cases, "direct" killing, i.e., an intentional killing, occurs, even though the body of the victim is in no way physically attacked. Acting directly against the body of another is therefore neither a necessary nor a sufficient condition for an intentional killing, and it is therefore not decisive in defining abortion, which is properly understood as the intentional killing, as a means or as an end, of a human being prior to or in the process of birth.

Finally, one could appeal to authority in arguing that removal of the embryo alone from the fallopian tube constitutes intentional abortion. Directive 45 of the Ethical and Religious Directives for Catholic Health Care Services (ERD), adopted by the U.S. bishops, states that "every procedure whose sole immediate effect is the termination of pregnancy before viability is an abortion." Directive 36 states, "It is not permissible, however, to initiate or to recommend treatments that have as their purpose or direct effect the *removal,* destruction, or interference with the implantation of a fertilized ovum."[15]

These directives do not settle the case because, unlike the earlier editions of the health care directives issued in 1954 and 1971, the current directives do not indicate which procedures constitute a "sole immediate effect of terminating a pregnancy." Does removal of the embryo from its pathological site of implantation fall under the norm prohibiting termination of pregnancy prior to viability? As Pope John Paul II indicated in *Evangelium Vitae,* the intrinsic wrongfulness of abortion consists in the *intentional killing* of an innocent human being as a means or as an end. Indeed, "termination of pregnancy" in the morally prohibited sense should be understood in this light. It is permissible to "terminate a pregnancy" by a variety of means. These actions include removal of a gravid cancerous uterus and removal of a fallopian tube with an obstructing fetus. These actions are not direct or intentional abortions, though they result in the death of a human being as an unfortunate side effect of a life-saving intervention. Direct abortion, "termination of pregnancy" in the morally illicit sense, is properly understood as the intentional destruction of human life—as a means or an end—prior to or in the process of birth, as stated before.

Imagine that a technique were found to facilitate transfer of an embryo from the fallopian tube to the uterus, and that the procedure were safe for both women and their developing children. If directive 45 or directive 36 were to be interpreted as condemning all removals in all situations, then these ectopic transplants would have to be forbidden in all Catholic hospitals. The embryo, who could easily be saved, would have to die because the life-saving transplantation would involve removing the embryo from its initial site of implantation, which is construed as an intrinsically evil act. This surely is not in accordance with the letter or spirit of the ERD. Since directives 45 and 36 were given to serve human life, not to undermine it, interpreting either directive to exclude all embryo transplantation in all circumstances would not accord with the goods that the directives are intended to serve.

Indeed, one could argue that the act of removal, considered by itself and independently of its effects, is a benefit for the embryo itself. The human embryo cannot properly develop in the fallopian tube, so removing the embryo from its pathological location is beneficial to the embryo, even if the later stages of a rescue attempt are virtually doomed to fail to produce a live birth. In removing the embryo from the fallopian tube, a pathological condition is alleviated for both the mother and the embryo, despite the unwanted side effect of virtually certain embryonic death.

In contrast, because uterine pregnancy in itself is not a pathology, to remove the embryo (or fetus) from the uterus prior to viability does not alleviate a pathological condition. Unlike tubal pregnancy, a uterine pregnancy considered in itself is simply not pathological for either the mother or the developing human being in utero. Directives 45 and 36 are best understood as addressing the case of uterine pregnancy, in which detachment from the uterus prior to viability is lethal to the child. The directives should not be understood to address the case of tubal pregnancies in which the embryo is removed from its pathological location.

Administration of Methotrexate (MXT)

MXT is a drug that inhibits cellular reproduction in rapidly growing tissue; it is also used to treat some forms of cancer, Crohn's disease, multiple sclerosis, psoriasis, and rheumatoid arthritis. In pregnancy, it can be used to inhibit reproduction of the rapidly dividing cells of the growing trophoblast (the forerunner to the placenta) and the embryo proper. MXT is currently considered by most physicians (including faithful Catholics, perhaps mistaken, but acting in good faith) as medically indicated and morally permissible to treat early tubal pregnancy due in part to its 82%–95% success rate.[16] Like removal of the embryo alone, MXT has the medical advantage of preserving the tube, thereby facilitating future fertility. In addition, its use is much less expensive,[17] not surgically invasive, and generally leads to faster recovery than surgery.

In practice, the use of MXT as medically indicated is in the vast majority of cases morally licit. MXT is not medically indicated for use if the fetal heart beat is detected because of its association with failure of treatment.[18] The vast majority of tubal pregnancies are diagnosed some 6–8 weeks into pregnancy, when the fetal heart beat can be detected.[19] So, if at 6–8 weeks no fetal heart beat is detected and hormone levels indicate a failed pregnancy, the embryo is no longer alive. MXT may be administered to arrest the so-called persistent ectopic pregnancy, that is, the continued growth of the trophoblast. In the rare case of a tubal pregnancy diagnosed prior to the point at which fetal heart beat is detectable (3.5 to 4 weeks postconception), is MXT acceptable?

Over the past decade, ethicists who accept that starting from conception, no human being should ever be intentionally killed, have debated the permissibility of using MXT to treat tubal pregnancy.[20] Arguments that the use of MXT to treat tubal pregnancy is intentional killing often mirror the arguments against removal of the embryo alone. From this perspective, the use of MXT in cases of tubal pregnancy is intentional killing because it leads to the death of the embryo "invariably" or with certainty, and it also seeks to affect the body of the embryo.

However, as noted in the previous section, neither the certainty of the effect nor the fact of acting upon the body of another entails that a lethal effect which follows from the action is intended.[21] Seventeenth century Jesuit Theophile Raynaud (1582–1663) asks us to imagine that we are fleeing on horseback from an unjust aggressor, and we find ourselves before a child playing on a narrow bridge. "Even though the child is not an unjust aggressor in this case, serious authors allow the horseman to continue his flight even if it means the death of the child."[22] In his flight, the horseman acts directly upon the child and does not act upon the child for the child's own good, yet the child's death or mutilation is still not intentional. Lethal contact with the body of another may still be a foreseen side effect of a morally permissible act.

Albert Moraczewski, OP, argues that the use of MXT constitutes not the intentional killing of the embryo but rather a healing act to prevent further damage to the fallopian tube, an act in which the death of the embryo happens to be a foreseen and regretful consequence. He writes, "The moral object is to stop the destructive trophoblast by stopping further protein synthesis; this is not achieved by killing the trophoblast or the embryo proper. Rather, death follows subsequently."[23] I tentatively agree with Moraczewski and others that use of MXT in treating tubal pregnancy is not intentional killing.[24]

One objection to this view is that the resolution of the ectopic pregnancy may very well take place by securing the death of the human embryo.[25] Moraczewski originally cautioned in 1996 that the effects of MXT must be verified prior to accepting its use because of uncertainty about whether resolution of the ectopic pregnancy resulted from death of the conceptus or from arresting of the growth of the trophoblast. The necessary data has not yet been provided. Moreover, the toxicology and teratology literature are replete with warnings that the drug is an abortifacient or causes birth defects. It may well be the case that MXT kills the embryo long before it resolves the trophoblastic hormonal activity. Thus, MXT secures a good end (saving the mother) via an evil means (killing the embryoblast, not the trophoblast).

This argument assumes that the chronological order of the effects determines whether that effect is intended, but this assumption is problematic. In the case of self-defense, the death of the attacker may come chronologically prior to the cessation of the attack, but that does not mean that self-defense is necessarily intentional killing. In a just war, a bomb dropped on a legitimate military target may have an explosion that first kills innocent civilians sleeping on a factory roof and then destroys the military target. But the bomber is not intentionally killing innocent civilians as a means to destroy the military target. As John Finnis, Germain Grisez, and Joseph Boyle point out:

> That a bad effect issues from an act more immediately and directly than a good effect, or precedes and causes a good effect, does not by itself make the bad effect a means to the good. A heroic soldier who throws himself on a grenade chooses to use his body as a shield so that the shrapnel will not kill his fellows. Yet he does not choose his own destruction as a means, even though the effect of throwing

himself on the grenade—his body's being destroyed as it absorbs or slows down the shrapnel—is more immediate and direct than, and indeed causes, the good effect of the grenade's doing little or no injury to his fellows.[26]

Even if MXT causes the death of the embryo prior to the end of trophoblastic activity, it does not follow that one necessarily chooses MXT as a means to cause the death of the embryo. It is true that one could choose MXT simply as a means to abortion. Similarly, one could choose removal of a gravid uterus simply as a means to abortion. Yet removal of a gravid uterus is not necessarily chosen as a means to abortion, as in the case of the gravid cancerous uterus when the removal is a means to save the woman with the death of the unborn accepted as a side effect. Likewise, choosing to treat ectopic pregnancy by means of MXT is not necessarily choosing abortion.

Using MXT to stop the ongoing damage to the fallopian tube by the trophoblast is an action that, considered by itself and independently of its effects, is not morally evil. This is evident from the acceptance, even by those who otherwise condemn the use of MXT, of using methotrexate to treat the so-called persistent ectopic pregnancy. In such cases, one may use MXT to stop the destructive action of the trophoblast upon the fallopian tube. As such, the use of MXT to stop the destructive activity of the trophoblast is ethically acceptable considered in itself and independently of its further effects.

Even if the use of MXT need not constitute intentional killing, some authors hold that it still violates the first condition of double-effect reasoning because it is a form of intentional mutilation. May writes that the trophoblast:

> is a vital organ of the unborn baby during gestation. Although it is discarded later on, it must be regarded as an integral part of the body of the unborn child. . . . One chooses to use MXT precisely because one knows that it will destroy the trophoblast, i.e., a vital organ of the unborn child. Its "therapeutic" effect is achieved only by means of its lethal effect on the unborn child. Moreover, the "therapeutic effect" does not benefit the unborn child but the mother and does so

only because of its nontherapeutic effect destroys the trophoblast of the unborn child, thus causing its death. . . . Even if the death is not precisely the means chosen, one cannot exclude from the means chosen the intentional violation of the bodily integrity of the unborn child and the causing of its death, and doing so, not for its benefit, but for the benefit of another.[27]

If one understands the trophoblast as a vital organ of the embryo, then it would seem that the use of MXT violates the first condition of double-effect reasoning because intentional mutilation of an organ is intrinsically evil.

Thus, the debate about the moral permissibility of MXT to treat tubal pregnancy hinges in part on whether its use is the "intentional mutilation of an organ," with the exact definition of each of these three major terms—"intentional," "mutilation" and "organ"—in dispute.[28] By "mutilation" I mean the intentional destruction or removal of an organ (or other vital body part) that inhibits the function that the organ has or will likely have in maintaining the health of the one possessing the organ. The removal or destruction must be intentional rather than a foreseen side effect of the action, because the foreseen side effects of an action do not define it. Removing body parts *simpliciter,* such as fingernail trimmings, is not mutilation because they are not vital parts, those necessary for the healthy functioning of the organism. Further, removing organs that do not currently but likely would inhibit health (e.g., a mastectomy upon discovery of precancerous growths) is also not mutilation.

Should the trophoblast be considered a vital organ of the embryo that is mutilated by MXT? There are considerations for and against considering the trophoblast as an organ of the embryo. The reasons to consider it as a vital organ include that the trophoblast shares the same DNA as the newly conceived human being; it does not share the DNA of the mother. Further, the fact that the trophoblast is shed at birth does not negate its consideration as a crucial part of the embryo; the same is true of baby teeth, which are truly parts of a human being that in later stages of maturity are discarded. In addition, some medical literature references identify the trophoblast as an organ.[29]

Other authors suggest that the placenta, and by implication the implanted trophoblast, should be considered an organ of both the mother and the human embryo or fetus.[30] Arthur Vermeersch holds that the "placenta is a common organ" to both the mother and the unborn child.[31] If the trophoblast and later placenta are considered to be organs of the mother also, then double-effect reasoning would seem to allow the MXT for the treatment of the mother's pathological organ—the trophoblast invading the fallopian tube. In other words, it would be considered a part of the mother impinging harmfully on another part of the mother.

Other considerations lead to the conclusion that the implanted trophoblast should not be considered an organ of the embryo. The ability of the trophoblast to survive the death of the embryo suggests that it may not be a part of the embryo's body. When an organism dies, the various vital organs of the organism—heart, liver, lungs, etc.—rapidly deteriorate unless artificially sustained. Human cells and organs can continue to survive only if placed in an artificial environment that mimics the natural context in which the cells or organs formerly thrived. In contrast, the trophoblast often continues its natural growth hours, days, and even weeks after the death of the embryo, without any artificial intervention. This suggests that the trophoblast is not simply a part of the embryo, in contrast to the heart, lungs, or liver of more mature human beings.

Further, as parts of a whole human body, organs have mutually beneficial actions for the good of the whole and each other (the heart pumps oxygenated blood from the lungs, which in turn receives the circulating blood from the heart). By contrast, the trophoblast, and later the placenta and umbilical cord, simply benefit the embryo. There is no "mutual benefit" typical of an organ, therefore the trophoblast would not seem to be simply a part of the embryo.

Finally, the fact that the embryo needs the trophoblast in order to survive does not demonstrate that it is a "vital organ" of the embryo. The embryo also needs the mother to survive, but she is not a vital organ of the embryo. The embryo needs atmospheric pressure within certain parameters in order to survive, but atmospheric pressure is not an organ of the embryo. The fact that the embryo and the trophoblast share DNA also does not indicate that the trophoblast is a vital organ, for many other parts of an organism (such as hair) share DNA but are not vital organs. If the trophoblast is not an organ of the embryo, then the argument fails that the use of MXT is ethically impermissible because it intentionally mutilates a vital organ.

However, for the sake of argument, let us assume that the trophoblast is an organ of the embryo. The question then becomes whether this is a case of intentional mutilation. The fact that MXT acts directly upon the trophoblast and not for the benefit of the trophoblast does not indicate that it is intentional mutilation. Cardinal Ioannes de Lugo, SJ, (1583–1660) argued that if an unjust aggressor uses an innocent child as a human shield, a person may defend himself against the attack by, for example, throwing a javelin through the human shield in order to kill the aggressor. Such an act, he held, is not intentional killing or intentional mutilation of the child.[32] As John Finnis, Germain Grisez, and Joseph Boyle point out: "In general, the fact that an act is done to (or 'upon') [person] X for the sake of [person] Y, or to Y for the sake of Y, provides no criterion for distinguishing between what is intended and what is accepted as a side effect."[33] In these cases (the tactical bomber, the horseman evading an attacker, and the human shield), damage is done against the body of an innocent person that is not for the benefit of this innocent person, yet this damage does not define the act but rather is a side-effect of an ethically legitimate act. If this reasoning is correct, then the ongoing damage to the tube caused by the trophoblast is a pathology that may be licitly treated by MXT.

On the other hand, several considerations suggest that the use of MXT may indeed be intentional mutilation by seeking to inhibit the normal growth of the trophoblast (albeit situated in an abnormal location). Following Michael Bratman and Thomas Cavanaugh, the following characteristics help distinguish intended effects from side-effects:[34] (1) the achievement of the effect presents a problem for the agent that occasions deliberation; (2) the achievement of the effect constrains other intentions of the agent; (3) the agent endeavors to achieve the effect, perhaps being forced to return to deliberation if circumstances change; and (4) the failure of the agent to realize the effect is a failure in the agent's plan.[35] If these characteristics are accepted, then inhibiting cellular reproduction in the trophoblast is intended. How to inhibit cellular reproduction is precisely the problem for the agent who deliberates how powerful a dose and at what frequency doses of MXT should be provided. The desired effect of MXT constrains the other intentions of the doctor, who must be careful not to prescribe any medications that will interfere with MXT's ability to inhibit cellular reproduction. The doctor endeavors to achieve the effect, perhaps being forced to adjust dosages if the desired effect does not transpire. Finally, it will be accounted a failure for the doctor prescribing MXT if the cellular inhibition does not take place. Given that the cellular inhibition is intended, is the use of MXT intentional mutilation?

As mentioned, mutilation might be defined as the intentional destruction or removal of an organ (or other vital body part) that inhibits the function that the organ has or will likely have in maintaining the health of the one possessing the organ. The inhibition of the cell divisions of the trophoblast would seem to fulfill this definition. However, since the embryo in the tubal pregnancy may be in the process of dying from other causes when the MXT is administered, it may be that MXT does not hasten the death of the fetus and therefore does not interfere with the function the organ has in promoting the health of the embryo.[36] Similarly, Dr. Alan Shewmon has argued that a severely injured person may be taken off life support, and once the dying process has begun, vital organs may be removed without hastening death and without this being considered intentional mutilation.[37] So, the permissibility of the use of MXT to treat tubal pregnancy may hinge on whether the MXT hastens death in a given case. If it does, this is a sign that mutilation has taken place.

These points are certainly debatable, and at this stage of the ethical conversation, the discussion about the permissibility of MXT has not reached a conclusion either through the consensus of ethicists or through an intervention from the Church's bishops or the papal Magisterium. I wish to emphasize again that in the vast majority of actual cases in which MXT is medically indicated, the death of the embryo has already occurred, so MXT cannot be construed as abortion in such cases.

One possible difficulty with this analysis is that the views expressed here about salpingostomy might conflict with what is said about MXT. If it were possible to remove the human embryo from the fallopian tube and implant it in utero, then wouldn't this option be not merely permissible but morally required, thereby excluding the permissibility of using MXT?

This difficulty is hypothetical, of course, because we do not currently have any reliable way of removing an embryo from the tube and placing it in the uterus. Even if this treatment were possible, in trying to save the life of the human embryo—or of any other human being—we need not make use of every treatment available in every circumstance. In each case, the burdens and benefits of the treatment must be considered, and treatments that are more burdensome than beneficial may be foregone. Salpingostomy may be permissible but is not obligatory.

Having examined the issue of ectopic pregnancy in some detail, what procedures should be permissible in Catholic hospitals? There is no debate about medical management or removal of the tube along with the embryo (salpingetcomy). Concerning the removal of the embryo alone while leaving the tube intact (salpingostomy) as well as the use of MXT, there remains a lively debate as to how to apply the principles widely accepted by those who defend the equal basic dignity of all human persons.

The theory of "probabilism" may be relevant for guiding action in these matters. When there are legitimate doubts about the application of a certain moral norm or about matters of fact, probabilism holds that one is free to form an opinion which according to "presentation of the facts or application of the law is probable, even if others hold an opposite and also probable opinion."[38] If probabilism is applied to these cases, until such time as that when the doubt about the issue has been removed, it would seem to follow that Catholic hospitals and physicians should be permitted to make use of all of the medical procedures discussed in this chapter: medical management, removal of the pathological tube containing the embryo, removal of the embryo alone, and the use of methotrexate.

Ectopic pregnancy is but only one kind of fetal surgery. In fetal surgery, a doctor may make many other interventions, some for the sake of the mother and others for the sake of the human being in utero. The ethics of other kinds of fetal surgery are relatively unexplored, but the next chapter examines a few cases in greater depth.

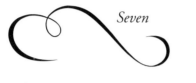

Seven

The Ethics of Fetal Surgery

The ethics of fetal surgery raise numerous questions. In this chapter, I would like to consider only three. Is the fetal human being a "patient," and if so, under what conditions? Why does the "reduction" of a twin pregnancy to one baby cause such difficulty for defenders of abortion? Is it morally permissible to prevent a dying fetal twin from bringing about the death or serious injury of a healthy fetal twin by means of umbilical cord occlusion? Perhaps the most prolific scholars exploring the ethical questions about fetal surgery are Frank A. Chervenak and Laurence B. McCullough. In a series of books and articles, they have established themselves as the foremost authorities in the area. How do they answer the first and fundamental question about fetal dignity? Chervenak and McCullough point out that there has been a long-standing debate about whether or not the human fetus has independent moral status.[1] Like many other debates, there has never been a definitive answer that has settled the matter once and for all to the satisfaction of all parties. Theological traditions disagree with each other and are often also internally divided. In a similar way, philosophy offers many different methodologies which lead to different conclusions about the issue, so reasonable people still disagree about whether the fetal human should be accorded basic human rights.[2] McCullough and Chervenak hold that the only rational course of action is to abandon the debate about whether or not the human fetus is a patient with independent moral status and to instead pursue a question that they think is answerable: Does the fetal human have dependent moral status? They write, "A philosophically more sound and clinically more useful line of ethical reasoning is that the moral status of the fetus depends on whether it is reliably expected later to achieve the relatively unambiguous moral status of becoming a child and, still later, the more unambiguous moral status of becoming a person. This is called the dependent moral status of the fetus."[3] According to McCullough and Chervenak's view, the human being in utero has dignity only when viable and when the pregnant woman presents herself to the doctor in order to secure help for the human fetus.

The proposal to shelve the debate about the independent worth and focus instead on the issue of dependent status faces a number of difficulties. First, the view of McCullough and Chervenak is self-defeating. They themselves presuppose a particular methodology, a methodology that is not universally accepted. So, if we ought to reject proposals that do not make use of a universally accepted methodology, we should reject their project. Second, the McCullough-Chervenak position rests on feigned neutrality. It is possible to be agnostic in theory about the value of human life in utero, but it is not possible to be agnostic in practice when one is treating fetal human beings. A physician treating a pregnant woman must either act as if the human being in utero is a second patient with independent worth or not. It is grossly irresponsible to "shelve" the question of the moral status of the fetal human when in fact a physician who is to treat a pregnant patient requesting medical intervention affecting the unborn must act in one way or the other. To decide to harm the fetal human being seemingly implies that the human fetus has no independent value, no matter what theoretical stance is taken on the question of fetal worth.

McCullough and Chervenak assert that the fetal human being has dependent status when and only when he or she is both viable and treatment is sought for him or her by the pregnant woman.[4] McCullough and Chervenak present no argument for the requirement of viability for moral worth. The thesis is simply asserted, the definition of viability is briefly explained, and then the conclusion is reasserted. In fact, viability—the ability to survive independent of the help of others—is irrelevant to moral status.[5] In cases of conjoined twins, one twin may be physiologically dependent upon the other, yet no one denies that both conjoined twins have equal basic dignity to each other and other persons. Furthermore, viability varies according to access to technology, but it is absurd to say that the moral worth of a person varies accord to one's proximity to a hospital. To live in one location rather than another is irrelevant for moral status. McCullough and Chervenak do give an argument for why the decision of the woman is relevant to whether or not the fetus is a patient: that independent moral status arises later and will not be possible without the decision of the woman to continue the pregnancy. "This is because the only link between a previable fetus and its later achieving moral status as a child, and then a person, is the pregnant woman's autonomy, exercised in the decision not to terminate her pregnancy, because technologic factors do not exist that can sustain the previable fetus ex utero. When the pregnant woman decides not to terminate her pregnancy and when the previable fetus and pregnant woman are presented to the physician, the previable fetus is a patient."[6]

This argument is unsound. It is false that the only link between a previable fetus and its later achieving moral status is the choice of the woman. If by "links" they mean a necessary (but not sufficient) condition, they are correct that a necessary condition for a child to have a second birthday is that the mother not abort him or her, but they are incorrect in claiming that this is the only condition. Other links understood in this sense include that the child does not die of natural causes prior to two years of age, that the child is not killed shortly after birth by someone else, and that a forced abortion is not performed, among many other links. If we understand the link of a woman's choice not to have an abortion as a sufficient condition for the child to achieve personhood, similar problems arise. Clearly, a woman can choose not to have an abortion, yet the child may die prior to birth during in involuntary miscarriage. Because Chervenak and McCullough's argument rests on a false premise, it does not justify their conclusion.

Chervenak and McCullough's treatment of fetal surgery is flawed in other ways as well. They write:

To protect the woman from being coerced, her husband or partner and other family members should be reminded that although they may have strong views for or against her participation, their role should be to support and respect the woman's decision-making process and its outcome. Their relationship to her is primarily one of obligation to respect and support her decision. Family members do not have the right to make decisions for her. When necessary, this aspect of the informed consent process should be made clear to family members. Clinical investigators should ensure that everyone involved in the consent process takes a strictly nondirective approach. Although not currently required in federal consent regulations, prospective monitoring of the consent process (e.g., in random sampling) could be used to enforce the nondirective approach.[7]

Chervenak and McCullough offer no justification for any of these controversial claims. It is true according to *Roe v. Wade* that the pregnant woman has the legal right to make the decision to abort. Whether or not she also has the moral right to fetal homicide remains a topic of vigorous disagreement. In *The Ethics of Abortion: Human Life, Women's Rights, and the Question of Justice,* I argue that there is no such moral right because there is a moral duty to refrain from abortion. Legally, there is no obligation whatsoever for family members, or anyone else for that matter, to refrain from voicing their opinions about her contemplated choice. At least in the United States, the First Amendment of the Constitution protects free speech rights, which are not rescinded in family relationships or when one takes the Hippocratic oath. From an ethical point of view, there is simply no obligation "to respect and support her decision," whatever that decision may be or to presuppose that all choices are ethically equal. If a decision is ethically permissible or commendable, then it should be respected and supported. If a decision is an ethically impermissible one, the decision should be neither respected nor supported. The person who makes the decision should be respected and supported as appropriate because all persons have dignity, but the decision itself warrants scrutiny. There is no ethical obligation to support and respect ethically wrong decisions such as the decision to drive under the influence of alcohol. Love and respect for others, including the potential drunk driver, demands that we seek ways to help a person avoid a wrongful choice, which in many circumstances includes trying to talk the person out of making a wrong decision. On a positive note, Chervenak and McCullough are correct in noting how fetal homicide impedes scientific research. "From the perspective of investigators, to obtain the cleanest results about outcomes for fetuses and future children, one would not want any pregnancies in which fetal surgery occurred to result in elective abortions."[8] In his article, "Fetal Therapy: Practical Ethical Considerations," Yves Ville makes the same observation: "However, owing to the high incidence of TOP [termination of pregnancy] following prenatal diagnosis of these conditions, comparative studies are going to be difficult to perform."[9]

In his discussion, TOP is a favored term, but this is unfortunate because "termination of pregnancy" is an ambiguous, inaccurate, and euphemistic phrase. It is ambiguous because vaginal birth, cesarean section, and spontaneous miscarriage also "terminate" a pregnancy. It is inaccurate because abortion can take place in cases where there is no "termination of pregnancy," such as committing selective abortion against one twin while leaving the other twin alive. It is euphemistic because termination of pregnancy—or better yet its acronym, TOP—sounds benign, innocent, and noncontroversial. The divisive reality is better conveyed by the more accurate, honest, and precise term: "abortion." Ville raises other ethical questions about fetal surgery. He notes a certain bias among practitioners of fetal surgery for suggesting treatments that may not be in the patient's best interest. "Offering treatment for a fetus demonstrating objective signs for an irreversibly poor outcome is questionable in that the benefit of treatment can be expected to be little if any and medical enthusiasm may also be strengthened with the view to improve one's own practice with the procedure."[10] A desire to strengthen one's surgical skills or pioneer new techniques may come into conflict with providing what is best for both patients: mother and child.

Ville also claims, "Prenatal diagnosis is the only field of medicine in which termination has a role in the management of a disease."[11] This claim is false because "termination" of a patient is not the management of a disease. As Jorge Garcia points out in his judicious discussion of physician-assisted suicide (PAS), to kill one is not to relieve his or her pain. Garcia's reflections can be extended to also show that killing is not management of a disease.

> Ending her pain cannot be a benefit to her for the usual reason, then, because here [in the case of PAS] the patient does not experience relief and thereafter live pain-free. As the end of her pain here does not improve her experience neither does it improve her life, her condition. Rather, she (her integrated human life) ends along with the pain, and *she* is in no condition at all during the period when she is lifeless. We cannot, then, meaningfully compare it with her condition over the same time had she lived. . . . Thus, it is difficult to see just what benefit our killing renders her, as it *improves* neither her experience, nor her life, nor her condition."[12]

Just as killing people to end their pain is not pain relief, so too is abortion not a management or cure of a disease. Indeed, if we define disease as a lack of proper biological functioning, to kill a fetus induces the maximum of disease: complete non-functioning.

Concerning the moral status of a human fetus, Ville writes, "Although the concept of the fetal status gaining more independence from its mother with gestational age is universally accepted, its importance is to be balanced with other issues including maternal safety as well as the severity of the fetal condition."[13] However, it is not universally accepted that a fetus's moral status is linked to his or her gestational age such that the more he or she develops physiologically, the greater the value the fetal human has. This gradualist or developmental view of the value of human life prior to birth is controversial and rejected by many people on a variety of grounds. For example, in tightly linking biological development to moral worth, the developmental view would seem to prove too much, that killing a thirteen-year-old is worse than killing a three-year-old. Obviously, those who oppose fetal homicide on the basis that all human life has equal basic value reject this view.[14] But many of the most prominent supporters of abortion, such as Peter Singer, Michael Tooley, David Boonin, and Judith Jarvis Thomson, also reject this view. Ville offers no argument for this view but simply assumes without justification that the developmental view is obviously true. Indeed, Ville's view of fetal status is inconsistent. He writes:

> The issue of fetal analgesia touches on the surgical approach itself in as much as on the "primum non nocere" principle in all procedures invasive to the fetus itself. It is well established that very preterm neonates experience pain and related autonomic neural connexions function from around 22 weeks of gestation. (Lee et al., 2005). It is therefore important that any directly invasive fetal procedure be preceded by appropriate fetal analgesia. . . . Practitioners who undertake termination of pregnancy at 24 weeks or later should also consider the requirements for fetal analgesia or sedation prior to fetocide before inducing labor."[15]

This approach is not consistent. If a fetal human being should not be harmed (*primum non nocere*), then it is true that this principle requires the use of analgesia for operations in which the human being in utero may suffer; but a fortiori, it is true that the more significant harm of death should not be inflicted on the fetal patient. The *primum non nocere* principle either applies to the unborn or it does not. This disjunction is also relevant in terms of twin pregnancies. The reduction of a pregnancy from twins to a single baby is controversial even among those who otherwise staunchly defend fetal homicide. In response to a *New York Times Magazine* story that raised the issue,[16] William Saletan's article in *Slate,* "Flaws in Pro-Choice Logic," points the spotlight squarely on the problem for defenders of abortion.[17] Why should defenders be troubled by an abortion that reduces a pair of twins to a single baby? They clearly are troubled, but they have a difficult time articulating why this is the case. Saletan recognizes the split thinking of many defenders of fetal homicide:

> Embryos fertilized for procreation are embryos; embryos cloned for research are "activated eggs." A fetus you want is a baby; a fetus you don't want is a pregnancy. Under federal law, anyone who injures or kills a "child in utero" during a violent crime gets the same punishment as if he had injured or killed "the unborn child's mother," but

no such penalty applies to "an abortion for which the consent of the pregnant woman . . . has been obtained." Reduction destroys this distinction. It combines, in a single pregnancy, a wanted and an unwanted fetus. In the case of identical twins, even their genomes are indistinguishable. You can't pretend that one is precious and the other is just tissue.[18]

Reduction of a pregnancy from twins to a single baby brings to the surface the usually implicit pro-choice double-think, causing cognitive dissonance.

One final question about fetal surgery is whether umbilical cord occlusion in cases of twin-twin transfusion syndrome is ethical.[19] In such cases, the twins are connected by a shared placenta. One of the twins is dying (for example, from imminent, irreversible cardiac failure), but the other twin is healthy. Once the first deteriorating twin dies, the other twin has a high risk of death or of permanent, serious neurological injury. Is it morally permissible to prevent the dying twin from causing the death or serious injury of the healthy twin by means of umbilical cord occlusion? Umbilical cord occlusion (UCO) is a procedure that cuts off the circulatory link between the twins but at the same time cuts off the life-supporting link to the placenta for the dying twin. The one action (UCO) brings about two effects: one good and life-saving, the other bad and life-terminating. Considering double-effect reasoning, the question is in part the following: Is UCO selective feticide, or is it a rescue of one twin at the expense of the foreseen but unintended death of the other?

Suppose for the sake of argument that the death of the weaker twin is not desired as a means or as an end in itself and that the fourth condition of double-effect reasoning is met, namely that there is a just cause for allowing the evil effect. My view in such a case is that the justification or condemnation of UCO depends on how the decision maker understands the distinction between intended effects and merely foreseen effects. If all certain or simultaneous effects of an action are intended, then UCO is impermissible according to double-effect reasoning. However, if one understands intended effects to be limited to what is chosen as a means or as an end—as part of one's plan or as a desired effect[20]—then UCO is permissible according to double-effect reasoning despite the certain and simultaneous negative effect of accelerating the death of the dying twin. According to double-effect reasoning, it is permissible not to prevent the foreseen death of one person in order to save the life of another. It is doubtless that fetal surgery gives rise to other ethical issues as well, but twin-twin transfusion syndrome is among the most difficult to evaluate. Without a cogent answer to our earlier questions about the ethical implications of fetal dignity in cases of reduction of pregnancy, the likelihood of coming to a just solution for cases of twin-twin transfusion syndrome is unlikely.

I hold that one person may not intentionally kill another person just because that other person has not yet been born. But this is obviously a controversial perspective. Thomson famously challenged this view by arguing that even if the human fetus has a right to live, the human fetus does not thereby have a right to make use of the body of his or her mother in continuing to live. Thus, according to Thomson's view, abortion is permissible even if the human fetus is a person and even if all human beings have intrinsic dignity. The next chapter examines various representations of and responses to objections to Thomas's famous violinist argument defending abortion.

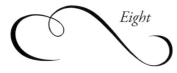

Eight

The Violinist Argument Revisited

The violinist analogy for defending abortion admits the basic human dignity of an unborn human being yet still justifies abortion. The argument begins with the picture of someone who wakes up to find himself hooked up as a source of life support for a famous violinist. It is held that he is justified in unplugging himself from the violinist, even though the violinist is a person. The analogy is then extended to the case of a pregnant woman, who, it is argued, may justifiably unplug herself from the fetal person. The principle involved in both cases is that the right to live does not include the right to make use of another person's body in order to live.

Though in theory *Roe v. Wade* professed agnosticism about when a conceptus may be said to become a human person, in practice the ruling denies fetal personhood. These denials have become less and less plausible both in terms of the scientific evidence that abortion kills a whole, living, unique, individual member of the human species and in terms of the moral discussion in which even staunch defenders of abortion, such as Frances Kissling, acknowledge that they are losing the debate.[1] In 2011,

Kissling made this startling admission on the front page of the *Washington Post:*

> In the nearly four decades since the Supreme Court ruled that women have a fundamental right to decide to have an abortion, the opposition to legal abortion has increased dramatically. Opponents use increasingly sophisticated arguments—focusing on advances in fetal medicine, stressing the rights of parents to have a say in their minor children's health care, linking opposition to abortion with opposition to war and capital punishment, seeking to make abortion not illegal but increasingly unavailable—and have succeeded in swinging public opinion toward their side. Meanwhile, those of us in the abortion-rights movement have barely changed our approach. We cling to the arguments that led to victory in *Roe v. Wade.* Abortion is a private decision, we say, and the state has no power over a woman's body. Those arguments may have worked in the 1970s, but today, they are failing us, and focusing on them only risks all the gains we've made.[2]

In her article "Rethinking *Roe v. Wade:* Defending the Abortion Right in the Face of Contemporary Opposition," Bertha Alvarez Manninen also admits that both public opinion and political tides have turned against *Roe v. Wade.*[3] She proposes to turn back the tide by revisiting the violinist argument. Manninen, following in the steps of Judith Jarvis Thomson, wants to defend the moral and legal right to abortion even if the human being in the womb is acknowledged to be a person from conception, a proposition that Thomson and Manninen both deny.

One of the chief objections to Thomson's violinist argument is sometimes called the "weirdness" objection. To be medically attached to some famous violinist is an utterly unrealistic, fantastic, and bizarre scenario, whereas pregnancy is familiar, natural, and utterly common. The more surreal the analogy, the less we are likely to rely on our intuitions for adjudicating actual cases.

Manninen seeks to remedy this difficulty by providing analogues to the violinist argument from actual cases. In the 1978 case of *McFall v. Shimp,* the Tenth Pennsylvania District Court ruled that no person should be forced to give up a kidney even in order to save another person's life. Manninen notes that "no person's right to life entailed that another person had to forcibly submit to unwanted bodily intrusion in order to sustain the former's life."[4] According to her view, defenders of unborn human life seek to establish that the unborn "possesses an *additional* right, *one that no other extra-uterine person possesses,* to be given whatever it needs for survival, including access to a woman's womb, regardless of whether she is willing to voluntarily provide it. . . . [T]here is no case (to my knowledge) in which one person's body was forcibly invaded in order to save another person."[5]

Manninen provides a Kantian argument for the conclusion that no person should be forced to surrender her body in order to aid another. "To compel a pregnant woman to submit to an unwanted intrusion of her body to sustain the life of the fetus violates her autonomous decision to do otherwise, and uses her body as a mere means to saving the life of the fetus."[6] Individual adults in need of blood transfusions, kidney transplants, or bone marrow donations are certainly persons, but other people are under no obligation to provide the needed aid, even if this means that the persons in need will die. Similarly, Manninen argues that even if it is conceded that the human being in the womb is a person with equal moral status to adults, pregnant women may still decline to allow their own bodies to be used in order to sustain fetal life.

However, if the human fetus is a person, this fetal person will also have the right to bodily integrity. The person in utero will likewise have the right not to be used simply as a means to realize someone else's desires, including the desire not to be pregnant and not to be a mother. The lethal violation of bodily integrity in abortion is a much more serious and irreversible loss than the partial violation of bodily integrity involved in donating a kidney or continuing pregnancy. Likewise, avoiding death is a more serious reason for allowing a side-effect than avoiding the difficulties of unwanted pregnancy. Indeed, the fetus has two goods at stake: bodily integrity and life itself. In normal cases of pregnancy, the woman does not. A fortiori, if people have a right to bodily integrity and so do not have a duty to donate a kidney, then people in utero have a right not to have their bodily integrity fatally violated through abortion.

No one should be forced to donate a kidney to save a human life, so it is even more obvious that no fetal person should undergo lethal violation of bodily integrity to save a woman from continuing to be a gestational/genetic mother. Indeed, the term "mother" is properly used for pregnant women. In his article "Manninen's Defense of Abortion Rights is Unsuccessful," Don Marquis notes:

> All mammals have mothers. A fetus is a mammal. Therefore, a fetus has a mother. Only the pregnant woman qualifies to be the mother of the fetus within her. All mothers are parents. All parents (unless exceptional circumstances obtain) have serious, special duties of care to their children. (Think here of your reaction to deadbeat dads.) Therefore, all pregnant women have serious, special duties of care to their children. Fetuses are children. Therefore, all pregnant women have serious, special duties to care for their fetuses."[7]

Regardless of whether or not the pregnancy was intended, parents have duties to their offspring. The duty of fathers to pay child support is evidence of this widely shared expectation.[8]

Alex Rajczi objects, "it is unclear that the father's potential sacrifices, over time, are equivalent to the intense sacrifices a mother must make over a nine-month period to carry a child to term."[9] Rajczi emphasizes the point even more strongly elsewhere: "We need to decide whether mothers have a duty to alleviate mortal needs created foreseeably but unintentionally—a duty that is strong enough to require her to sacrifice her body for nine months, etc."[10] Likewise, Manninen believes a pregnant woman "completely surrender[s] the use of her body, even if doing so goes against her will, for nine months."[11]

These kinds of descriptions unrealistically and unfairly exaggerate what happens to a woman's body during pregnancy.[12] It is not that the woman completely sacrifices her body or loses control of her body for nine months, as if she were in a prison camp or having continual epileptic seizures for thirty-eight weeks. An expectant mother does not have symptoms of advanced Parkinson's disease; she is not in a coma. Indeed, during the beginning of pregnancy and sometimes even later into pregnancy, a woman may not even be aware that she is carrying a baby. The language used by defenders of abortion of "complete sacrifice" describes accurately, however, what happens to the fetal person who gives up use of his or her body not partially for nine months, but completely and forever.

How much pain, effort, and struggle is involved in pregnancy, and how does this compare to the sacrifices demanded of fathers?[13] The answer varies from mother to mother and from father to father, but we can estimate the average amount of sacrifice in financial terms. In his "Surrogate Mother Case," Rajczi estimates the cost to the gestational mother for pregnancy and placing the child for adoption at $100,000. In point of fact, in the United States, "surrogate mothers are typically paid $15,000."[14] Do we then require less of fathers than we do of expectant mothers? In the U.S., the average amount of child support paid by fathers is $4,243 per year or more than $89,000 until age twenty-one.[15] Measured in average financial terms, the father has provided more support for the child than the expectant mother after just four years. Of course, any minimally morally decent father must do much more than provide a check each month, as must any minimally morally decent mother. Most especially, neither parent should ever intentionally harm their own child or even allow a foreseeable but preventable harm, save for the most serious moral justifications.

When defenders of the violinist argument such as Rajczi and Manninen speak of the "right to decide what happens in and to one's body," what exactly does the term "right" mean? The equivocality of the term "right" in the abortion debate was pointed out long ago by John Finnis, who utilizes the work of Wesley Hohfeld to disambiguate the term.[16] A Hohfeldian "liberty right" to have X is the claim that the agent has no duty *not* to have X. For example, if a person has a right to free speech, this means that the person has no legal or ethical duty to refrain from speaking. In contrast, if a person has a "claim right," then *other* people have a duty to aid, provide, or do something or refrain from doing something with respect to the person with that right. An agent's right to live is a claim right, which means that other people have a duty not to intentionally kill the agent.

How do these various kinds of rights apply to abortion? Consider abortion understood as a claim right. All people have duties not to interfere with other people's bodies. This duty readily connects to the violinist analogy because doctors have duties not to hook up unconsenting people to violinists. Hopkins notes that "the fetus has no right to occupy its mother's (or anyone else's) body."[17] So, does the fetal person violate the claim rights of women to control their bodies?

People do indeed have a duty not to occupy the body of other persons. But a human fetus, like a human newborn or a human adult with a serious mental handicap, has no duties, so the supposition that the "fetus has no right to occupy its mother's body" is false. Winds, water, or animals cannot violate someone's rights because these beings have no duties in virtue of not being capable of acting knowingly and freely. So too, it is literally impossible for any human fetus, any human newborn, or any human adult with a serious mental handicap to violate anyone's claim rights. Therefore, abortion cannot be justified in terms of a mother's claim right against her unborn child or the child's lack of a right or duty not to occupy the mother's body.

On the one hand, the "right to control one's body" could itself be understood as a liberty right. A right to control what happens in and to one's body may be understood to mean (analytically) that the agent has no duty to refrain from an abortion. But if the right to control one's body is understood in this sense, then the assertion of this right to justify abortion is question begging because precisely what is at issue is whether or not there is a duty to refrain from abortion. If we assert a "right to control one's body" understood in this sense, then the question of whether abortion is permissible remains unanswered.

Perhaps the "right to control one's body" should be understood as a premise in an argument to justify the conclusion that abortion is permissible. However, the right to control what happens in and to one's body admits many exceptions, both legally and morally. This right does not include the right to take heroin for fun, the right to undress in public, or the right to shout fire in a crowded theatre. So, taken as a universally true premise without exceptions, there simply is no such thing as the right to control what happens in and to one's body. This premise cannot be used to justify abortion.

A third problem with justifying abortion via a liberty right to control one's body involves the rights of the fetal person. All human persons have claim rights to not be intentionally killed. But if the human fetus is a person, he or she also has a claim right not to be killed. I say "he or she" deliberately, for it is a matter of biology that every human fetus is either male or female, and, on the supposition of the violinist argument, the human fetus is not an "it" but a person, a "he" or a "she." If we grant the supposition of the violinist argument, a liberty right to intentionally kill the human fetus cannot exist, because the claim right of the unborn child not to be killed means that all other people have a duty not to intentionally kill the fetal person. So, the claim right to life of the fetal person means that there is no liberty right to abortion, where abortion means intentionally killing the human being prior to birth as a means or as an end.

For this reason, the case of donating a kidney is significantly different from the case of abortion. In the case of donating the kidney, you foresee that the sick person will die unless you donate a kidney. In not donating a kidney, no one's right to life is violated because the person dies from the underlying illness. In contrast, in the abortion case, the fetus's right to life is violated because the abortion intentionally kills the fetus. Recall, too, that the violinist analogy concedes that the human fetus is a person with the same basic rights as other persons. If so, then the human fetus also has a right to decide what happens to and in her own body—a right to bodily integrity. Now, the fetus, like an unconscious adult, cannot decide anything, but if the right to bodily integrity is to have any significance, it must mean that other people cannot violate your body by tearing out your organs and dismembering you without your consent. But this is precisely what takes place to the fetus in typical abortions. So the intuition that one should not be forced to undergo surgery to remove one's kidney a fortiori supports the conclusion that the human fetus should not be subject to the even greater bodily violation of abortion.

In response, Thomson's argument could be construed as defending the view that abortion ought not to be understood as intentional killing but rather as removing the developing person with the side-effect of fetal demise. Thomson is defending not termination abortions but only evacuation abortions with the foreseen but not intended death of the unborn.

Thomson may indeed be defending only the foreseen death of the unborn. If so, she has provided no defense of the reality of abortion as practiced. Abortion has the intention of ending the life of the human being in utero. For this reason, when the baby survives the abortion, it is accounted as a "botched" or "attempted" abortion, a failure of what was intended. Indeed, sometimes when the baby is born alive, the practicing physician will kill the child. For example, the Associated Press reported, "A doctor [Kermit Gosnell] whose abortion clinic was described as a filthy, foul-smelling 'house of horrors' that was overlooked by regulators for years was charged Wednesday with murder, accused of delivering seven babies alive and then using scissors to kill them."[18] Later in pregnancy, following viability, where there is indeed a choice between removing the baby alive or dead, the abortion is done to secure the death of the child. The same intention to kill is true of many women who choose abortion. In his article "Can Technology Fix the Abortion Problem? Ectogenesis and the Real Issues of Abortion," Patrick Hopkins notes that for many women:

> What is most important about the right to have an abortion in the first place is that one could avoid "having a child," *not* that one could avoid *pregnancy*. A situation in which pregnancy could be ended but the fetus still grew into "their" child somewhere else would not suffice. What was most important was that there not be a child who was "theirs" at all. In fact, for many who hold this position, *their first choice would be to kill the fetus; their second choice would be to continue the pregnancy and keep the child; their last choice would be to give the fetus up for adoption.* Typically, the reason given is that it would be an unacceptable emotional burden to know that "my" child was somewhere "out there."[19]

Surely this desire to kill one's offspring ought not to be gratified. There are men with similar desires, desires that could only be satisfied by killing the child. In some cases, a man will have created a new human being with a woman who does not share his desire to not care for the child and so the woman refuses to get an abortion. For men, the right to gratify the desire not to continue to be a genetic parent does not justify abortion because this would interfere with the bodily integrity of the mother, and it would also justify infanticide. Indeed, the "right not to be a genetic parent" exercised after one has already become a genetic parent, leads to a denial of the right to life of even adult children. Of course, if the fact that the child is a person voids the right to relinquish being a genetic parent, then adult children as well as fetal children ought not to ever be intentionally killed by their parents or anyone else. In any case, the physician's intention to kill, and sometimes the mother's, renders Thomson's defense of forcseen but not intended fetal demise irrelevant to abortion as it is practiced.

Finally, Dennis O'Brien argues that the reality of pregnancy—the unique, intimate relationship between the human being in utero and the pregnant woman—changes the ethics of feticide: "The pregnant woman's womb is not just a geographic location for an independent entity that would be the same if it were located someplace else."[20] To deny this reality is to reduce the pregnant woman to a "container."

The intimacy argument, as articulated by O'Brien, raises an important question: Why should independent *moral* status require independent *physical* status? We don't think that one conjoined twin may licitly or legally authorize a third party to kill his conjoined brother in order to terminate their intimate relationship. Indeed, the intimate relationship that always exists in pregnancy is a powerful argument *against* abortion. Relationship is precisely the correct word, for in pregnancy there is a relationship between two persons: an expectant mother and her own dependent child. One cannot have an intimate relationship with a thing. Sound ethical reasoning and just laws hold that human mothers and fathers have serious duties to care for and, above all, not harm their own dependent progeny. So, the intimate relationship that exists in every pregnancy gives rise to the duty of the mother to not harm her own child prior to or after birth, including by ending the child's life. Precisely because an expectant woman is a mother rather than a mere container, she has duties to her dependent unborn child.

The latest versions of the violinist argument fail, but there will doubtless be sequels. Thomson's argument is that one person (the woman) may intentionally kill another person (the fetus) under certain circumstances (if the pregnancy is too burdensome). This principle also finds application at the end of life where it is held by some that it is ethically permissible for one person (the doctor) to kill another person (the sick or dying) in certain circumstances (informed consent to die). This topic—physician-assisted suicide—is the subject of the next chapter.

Nine

Faith, Reason, and Physician-Assisted Suicide

Disputes about the dignity of the human person tend to cluster around the beginning of life and end of life. Earlier chapters have addressed several beginning-of-life issues, and the next three chapters address end-of-life issues. This chapter addresses two challenges to the view that suicide (including physician-assisted suicide) is ethically impermissible, a violation of the dignity of the human person and natural law. H. Tristram Engelhardt challenges, not the prohibition of suicide itself, but the justification of this prohibition in terms of the natural law, while David Thomasma challenges an absolute prohibition on suicide based on the example of Christ and the martyrs.

In his essay "Physician-Assisted Suicide Reconsidered: Dying as a Christian in a Post-Christian Age," Engelhardt rightly points out that the revelation of God in both New and Old Testaments, as well as the tradition of the Church, leads one to conclude that physician-assisted suicide is morally wrong. He argues persuasively that the Fathers and Councils of the Church speak against suicide as a natural extension of the Christian attitude towards life, suffering, and death.[1] These attitudes, insights, and doctrines are summarized and crystallized in Roman Catholic theology through the authoritative pronouncement of John Paul II in *Evangelium Vitae*. He writes:

> *I confirm that euthanasia is a grave violation of the law of God,* since it is the deliberate and morally unacceptable killing of a human person. This doctrine is based upon the natural law and upon the written word of God, is transmitted by the Church's Tradition and taught by the ordinary and universal Magisterium.[2]

This pronouncement meets the requirements laid down in the Vatican Council II document *Lumen Gentium* for infallibility.[3]

David Thomasma's "Assisted Death and Martyrdom" would likewise seem to be an appeal to theological authority, namely the authority of the martyrs. St. Sebastian, Thomasma argues, sought his own death, as did St. Perpetua. Sebastian requested and indeed commanded his own troops to carry out their orders to kill him. Similarly, Perpetua aided the gladiator who was summoned to kill her. According to Thomasma:

> She guides his hand to her throat to help him. This assistance in her own dying, this treasuring of her martyrdom for Christ, led the narrator/observer to comment: "Perhaps it was that so great a woman, feared as she was by the unclean spirit, could not have been slain had she not herself willed it."[4]

The example of both Sebastian and Perpetua would seem to call into question the Church's teaching on assisted suicide. They both sought out aid in death, yet are both honored in the tradition as saints and martyrs. In fact, they were doing nothing more than what every Christian is called to do: imitate the example of Jesus Christ.

Is it really plausible, however, to suggest that Jesus himself committed suicide? Although Jesus did not commit suicide in the fullest sense of the term insofar as his death did not follow from his own hand, the status of the death of Christ is far from clear according to Thomasma. Thomasma argues that Jesus's death, though not without ambiguity, was in fact a form of self-killing.

> Jesus did, in fact, fulfill part of a definition of suicide, the elements of both willing one's own death, and putting into action a plan to bring it about. There is an active intent and plan in Jesus's mission, that is missing in those who think we should shun willing and acting to bring to pass our own death or the death of another.[5]

According to this view, Jesus willed His own death. That is, He committed an act that can rightly be described as suicide. Far from considering Christ's death a "special case" in light of His role in salvation, the martyrs "imitated Christ's death and through that imitation considered their deaths a gain."[6] Hence, insofar as Christians are called to imitate Christ, there would seem to be a "Christian case" for physician-assisted suicide. Relying as it does on the authority of the example of Christ and the martyrs, Thomasma's argument in favor of physician-assisted suicide would, if cogent, be most powerful in the theological sphere.

However, there exists a conflict among theological authorities. Church tradition unanimously condemns suicide, but the example of the martyrs and Christ suggest suicide may sometimes be justified. If theology proper follows from the revelation of God, how does the theologian resolve the difficulty? Clearly, there is no single answer to this question. In terms of Catholic and Orthodox theology, the reading of Scripture takes place within an interpretative tradition, and insofar as any reading cannot be reconciled with this tradition, the reading is to that extent problematic. Having already established from the perspective of the Christian tradition that suicide is an act that is incompatible with living new life in Christ, if we also believe in the impeccability of Jesus, then these considerations raise doubts about Thomasma's interpretation of Christ's death.

These doubts are warranted. I believe that the error of Thomasma's interpretation arises from failing to distinguish between suicide as choosing one's death as a means or as an end, and martyrdom as allowing one's death for the sake of some higher good. Christ did not choose His own death as a means or as an end. He knew He would die and allowed this to take place rather than disobey His Father's will. In the Matthean account of the agony in the garden (Matt. 26:39–44), three times Jesus prays to avoid embracing the suffering of Good Friday. "My Father, if it is possible, may this cup be taken from me. Yet not as I will, but as you will." In these passages, Jesus does not seem to be seeking out His death. There is certainly no sense that He holds His death to be a good. Rather, Christ submits to the Father's will by allowing or accepting His place as a suffering servant. As St. Anselm of Canterbury suggests in *Cur Deus Homo:*

> God did not, therefore, compel Christ to die; but he suffered death of his own will, not yielding up his life as an act of obedience, but on account of his obedience in maintaining holiness; for he held out so firmly in obedience that he met death on account of it.[7]

In the economy of salvation, God commands not Christ's death but Christ's obedience. As a side effect of this intended obedience, Christ is put to death. Just as a general may fully foresee that his troops will die in an invasion yet not intend for his troops to die, so too Jesus's death was foreseen but not intended in the Father's plan. To say otherwise is to endanger the justice of God, making God into a retributive Being who takes his vengeance out on an innocent victim. Likewise, Jesus, by perfectly conforming to the will of the Father, fully foresaw but did not intend His own death.

Both Jesus's words and deeds manifest a foreknowledge and acceptance of death, but they do not indicate that He sought out or chose death. In accepting his fate, Jesus does not run away when Judas comes with the elders to arrest Him, but He does not rush out to meet them either. Likewise at His trials, Jesus's stance towards His judges, accusers, and tormentors is almost entirely passive. He accepts His place but does not choose or "actively" bring about His death. This is why Scripture speaks of Jesus as laying down His life rather than taking His own life (John 10:11).

Jesus did clearly plan and foresee that He would die. But although He knew that He would die and did not prevent this outcome from taking place, this stance of the will is to be distinguished from intending or choosing to die. The difference then between suicide and martyrdom is found in the distinction between, on the one hand, choosing death as a means for whatever end and, on the other hand, foreseeing or permitting death to avoid giving up some other good (e.g., moral integrity, salvation, or obedience to the Father). There is a world of difference, therefore, between the deaths of Jesus and Judas. As a sign of love, Christ made Himself vulnerable even unto death despite foreseeing the pain. After his betrayal, Judas became desolate and then hanged himself, presumably to avoid the pain. Jesus was the archetype of the martyr; Judas was the archetype of the suicide.

Hence, although He fully foresaw His death, Christ did not properly will, intend, or choose His death as does a person who commits suicide. Because Christ did not commit suicide, the appeal to the example of martyrs as parallel to those who request physician-assisted suicide is considerably weakened. Even if Thomasma's interpretation of the stories of Sebastian and Perpetua is correct, it would seem that, despite their good intentions, their reasoning was mistaken. Such erroneous interpretations of the mind of Christ are sadly not unusual in the Christian tradition, which is made clear by the call of John Paul II in *Tertio Mellenio* to repent for such historical mistakes as the crusades and inquisitions. Just as various figures in the Old Testament sometimes commit what might be called "material wrongdoing" and are nevertheless figures deserving of respect and honor, so too the saints and martyrs following the period of the New Testament are not immune from intellectual and moral errors, despite their good intentions.

Insofar as Thomasma's "Assisted Death and Martyrdom" rests its argumentative weight upon the authority of the martyrs, his essay makes a fundamentally theological argument. I believe this argument fails theologically because his interpretation of the death of Christ jars with authoritative readings of Scripture. However, this theological failure may be clarified by ethical reasoning that does not appeal to premises supplied solely by revelation. Philosophy can help us answer the following questions that naturally arise in the context of distinguishing suicide from martyrdom: Why is suicide morally different from martyrdom? How is choosing death different from fully foreseeing yet not preventing death? Or more generally, how significant is the distinction between intending some bad effect and foreseeing but not preventing it?

We can recognize the importance of distinguishing intention from foresight when considering common cases. The intention of a professor who regrettably foresees that he or she will bore students is surely better than that of a professor who sets out to bore students.[8] We can foresee that people will die in car crashes whenever a freeway is built, but this differs from building a freeway in order to kill people. A government that accepts foreseen harm to community health by allowing the use of alcohol differs from a government that introduces these substances to a given population precisely to harm the citizens. The Anglo-American legal system reflects these common-sense intuitions by distinguishing between intended and merely foreseen harms. In sum, if the distinction between intention and foresight does not have moral importance, then many common-sense moral and legal assumptions will require extensive revision. In his article, Thomasma has given us no reason to doubt the moral importance of the distinction.

A defense of the distinction between intention and foresight does not need to rely solely upon intuitions, no matter how common, how strong, or how deeply presupposed by legal tradition. We can in fact make a philosophical case for the distinction.[9] I suggest a Thomistic defense of it. Morality is about *human actions*—that is, actions that follow from reason and will—and not about *the acts of human beings*—that is, actions (such as indigestion and sleep walking) that "happen" to human beings involuntarily. Human action, as Aquinas explains in *Summa Theologiae* I-II, questions 6–17, involves seven (or, if there exists a plurality of means, nine) interlocking acts of knowing and willing. Human action begins with understanding or foresight of possible happenings (*intellectus*) and proceeds through willing (*voluntas*), enjoyment (*frui*), intention (*intentio*), sometimes deliberation (*consilium*) and consent (*consensus*), choice (*electio*), command (*imperium*), and use (*usus*). Before considering how the process of human action clarifies the importance of the intention/foresight distinction, an example may illuminate how this process unfolds.

Human action begins with knowledge of what could take place—take, for example, the building of the atomic bomb. One foresees (*intellectus*) a possible outcome. Having been told by scientists that it was possible to build such a weapon, President Roosevelt considered whether or not this possibility was attractive. He became attracted to the possibility of making a bomb because it could be of great use in the war. This stage of Roosevelt's human action may be called an act of willing (*voluntas*). He recognized not only that the proposed end could come about (*esse*) but also desired this end as good (*sub ratione boni*). Sometimes, the process of human action proceeds no further. An agent simply recognizes some possibility, recognizes it as a good, and takes no further interest in it. In this case, however, the president "took delight" (*frui*) in the possibility of having such a good. "Such a weapon would be able to end the war much more quickly." If our attraction, or "entertaining," of the project does not end at this stage but rather leads to the point where we move to realize the end in question, then we may speak of intention (*intentio*).

Roosevelt, of course, decided to build the bomb. He formed an intention to accomplish this end. A question naturally arose: How am I to bring about this goal? This stage of human action corresponds to deliberation (*consilium*). If one is to attempt to develop a technological breakthrough such as the atomic bomb, there are many options as to how to go about it. One could hold international symposia and bring all the world's experts together to openly exchange information and collaborate on the project, as now takes place in the quest for a cure for AIDS. The president ruled out this option at once, giving consent (*consensus*) to one of the other means available, namely secret research undertaken by the best scientists available and underwritten by the government. Next, he made the choice (*electio*) that this was indeed the route to be taken. In order to follow through with this decision, Roosevelt exercised presidential privileges and issued directives to various government and military officials to conduct research and experiments. Aquinas designates these stages of human action as command (*imperium*) and use (*usus*). *Usus* is the very nexus in which the internal desires and reasoning of the agent come together with the (sometimes) external movements towards the desired and reasoned effects.[10]

The progression of the nine stages indicates an increasing commitment of the person to the end in question. An agent who recognizes that he or she could, in a certain case, steal (*intellectus*) is not as committed to that end as one who is attracted to theft (*voluntas*) and further entertains (*frui*) the thought of achieving the end of stolen loot. The one who decides to steal (*intentio*) but does not actually choose the means to achieve this end (*electio*) is, again, less committed to the theft than an agent who deliberates and actually follows through with the theft (*executio*). Thomas writes:

> Consider when someone wants to do something for a good or an evil end, and on account of some impediment stops; another person however continues the motion of the will until the work is complete. It is clear, that the will of this kind is more firmly committed to good or evil, and in this respect worse or better.[11]

In other words, Aquinas's stages of human action help to evaluate the extent to which an agent is committed to an end, be it good, bad, or indifferent. If death is an evil, then the agent who chooses death identifies himself with this evil to a much greater extent than one who foresees but does not prevent or intend death.

Of course, not to prevent one's foreseen death can, in certain circumstances, be an evil act. Consider, for example, foolhardy acts such as "playing chicken" in automobiles. Deaths resulting from these foolish displays of bravado are not intended, but they are nevertheless blameworthy. However, sometimes one is faced with the choice of *either* sinning *or* being killed. In such cases, it is meritorious to refuse to sin despite fully foreseeing that one will be killed as a result. This is precisely the choice of the martyr—to accept death as a foreseen side effect of the choice to be faithful.

However, even if one's intention makes a difference in distinguishing the nature of the act one is performing, is not intending one's own death sometimes itself a good? Does not the rule forbidding suicide arise from an anthropomorphic view of the Deity whose authority and boundaries we irrationally fear to trespass?[12] Can we not reinterpret the application of such rules in light of the relevant human goods? To answer these questions, which are raised at least implicitly in Thomasma's contribution, requires a word about the function of law and the ascription of death as a good for the human person.

According to Aquinas, God aids the human person in his or her return to God through grace, which strengthens the weakened will, and
through law, which enlightens the darkened intellect. All laws given by
God, certainly the Decalogue and even the dietary laws of the Jews, do
nothing more than help an agent to understand what acts are to be pursued and what acts are to be avoided.[13] Rules, then, save for those few
regulations that fall under positive law, such as appointed times of fasting,
do not make an act right or wrong. To ask questions about making exceptions to rules[14] is to misunderstand the function of rules, as if rules made
an action wrong rather than merely reflected the wrongness of an action
and as if we could merely adjust or suspend the rule, thereby changing
the nature of what we are morally doing.

The articulation of the difference between Thomasma's implicitly
voluntaristic conception of law and Aquinas's explicitly rational conception of law—found in *Summa Theologiae* I-II, questions 90–108—is profound. In the voluntaristic understanding of ethics, we have a divine
voluntarism which proposes rules through Church tradition. The task of
the moral theologian is then the task of a lawyer who applies the laws in
the books to particular cases, arguing about the intent of the law giver
and interpreting the law in such a way as to secure the desires of the cli-
ent. The lawyer-theologian is on a quest for a possible justification for
suspending, altering, or reinterpreting the rule. On the other hand, according to the natural law account advocated by Aquinas, the human
person has a created nature and is guided in fulfilling his or her nature by
grace aiding the will and by law aiding the intellect. God's law, or Church
tradition, does not make something right or wrong but merely informs
us that something is right or wrong independently of any positive law.
A moral theologian helps to determine which acts, given the nature of the
human person and his or her destiny, are conducive to this final end. The
moral theologian is somewhat akin to a doctor who articulates what in reality is conducive to being healthy through various "rules" such as "don't
smoke." Tampering with the rule does nothing to change the reality.

Within this rationalist, rather than voluntarist, perspective and given
also Aquinas's conception of the human person, it becomes clear why the
moral norm against suicide of all kinds aids the human person on this

quest to union with God in love. The Old Testament, as Thomasma help-fully notes, suggests certain themes about death. He writes:

> [The first is that] death is an evil not originally intended by God for human life (the Garden of Eden story). The second is that death is due to human responsibility for stepping over our own boundaries as defined by being a creature, one created by God with both power and limits (the story of Cain and Abel). The third is that death is a result of sin (through Adam came sin, and through sin, death—St. Paul).[15]

Why would the Old Testament portray death in this way? From the philosophical perspective advocated by Augustine and continued in Aquinas, evil is understood as a lack of due perfection. Insofar as life is a perfection of the human person—indeed, a perfection presupposed by all other human perfections such as knowledge, health, eyesight, and friendship—lacking the perfection of life is an evil. The Old Testament presents life as a good.

Thomasma contrasts the Old Testament, with its emphasis on creation, with the New Testament's spiritual emphasis. He writes:

> [T]he New Testament offers alongside the Old a different and contrasting view of death that also feeds into the rule against killing. It may provide some possible justification for suspending the rule. . . . On this view, while death is an ontological evil for personal bodily identity, it is a spiritual good because it brings about the maturing of the Christian into a new life. Death may be a good then, and intending or willing it may be a virtue.[16]

According to this view, death is an evil for the human body but a good for the person as the necessary conduit to new and eternal life in God. Insofar as death is a good, like other goods, it may be licitly chosen or intended as a means or an end.

One can detect here, I believe, two philosophical mistakes. The first is the lack of requisite conceptual distinctions between good and evil. The fact that some evil brings about some good or some good brings about some evil does not change the nature of evil into good or good into evil.

Let us say that I am tortured by captors from whom I eventually escape. Following my escape, I become a more loving, generous, and sensitive person. It does not follow that because good resulted from my experience that torture and imprisonment are goods for my captors or me. The forgiveness of sins is a great good, and forgiveness of sins comes about only because of sin, but we certainly cannot conclude from these observations that sin itself is a good. In a similar way, we cannot reason that because eternal life is a great good, and death brings about eternal life, that death is a good. Although many evils may be connected with life (such as severe pain, debilitation, or sickness), these evils must all be distinguished from life. That is, just because an evil such as sickness is found in conjunction with a good such as life does not mean that sickness is a good or life is an evil.

The second philosophical mistake is a Cartesian separation of body and soul. Death, it is argued, is ontologically evil for the body of a person but good for the "Christian [person brought] into a new life." Human persons, however, are a unity of body and soul. Since human beings are not pure spirits merely using or possessing their own bodies but rather *are* their bodies (though not, of course, merely their material bodies), what is evil for the human body is evil for the human person. Since death is not a good for the human body, but rather a privation of a due good, intending or willing death is not a good for the human person. Hence, in an ethics in which one is to want and seek the good for oneself and others (i.e., to love your neighbor as yourself), intentional killing of human beings has no place.[17]

In contrast to Thomasma's revision of the classic Christian position on suicide, Engelhardt's "Physician-Assisted Suicide Reconsidered: Dying as a Christian in a Post-Christian Age"—which reaches sound conclusions, often by sound reasoning from revealed premises—seems to err in distinguishing "Christian theology" from "secular philosophy" or unaided reason as if the two were natural enemies. This mistake makes his case against physician-assisted suicide less powerful than it could be.

Disagreements between Catholics and other Christians about the role of philosophy in theology may seem intractable, but let me list a few reasons why I believe that Engelhardt's proposed sharp dichotomy between faith and reason (i.e., secular philosophy) fails. First, Christian revelation seems to support the idea that one can learn moral truths without the aid of explicit revelation. Second, theology does not determine all philosophical questions, hence philosophy and theology are not in these respects even potential rivals. It is only in certain overlapping areas that apparent conflicts arise. Third, at least implicitly, a theology almost always presupposes a philosophy, suggesting that strong claims of incompatibility between the two are mistaken. Fourth, practically speaking, philosophy has proven helpful in removing objections to Christian moral belief. Finally, philosophy has offered reasons in support of Christian moral belief. For these reasons, one cannot sustain an easy opposition between faith and reason, between theology and philosophy, or between sacred and secular learning.

Each of these five points merits further consideration. First, Engelhardt's implicit fideism does not accord well with revelation. Both the Old and New Testament writers seem to indicate that one may learn truths revealed by God through the use of natural reason. Some stories seem simply to presuppose this view. For instance, Cain killed Abel before the revelation of the Ten Commandments. However, there is no explicit record of God "telling" Cain that fratricide was immoral. Yet Cain, as his reaction testified, did in fact know that what he did was wrong. How did he come to this knowledge? Cain knew this truth without revelation. In other words, Cain recognized the illicit nature of fratricide through the use of his own conscience formed by the light of natural reason, the law "written on the human heart" (Rom. 2:14–16). Likewise, in the New Testament, we read in Romans 1:18–20:

> The wrath of God is being revealed from heaven against all the godlessness and wickedness of men who suppress the truth by their wickedness, since what may be known about God is plain to them, because God has made it plain to them. For since the creation of the world God's invisible qualities—his eternal power and divine nature—have been clearly seen, *being understood from what has been made,* so that men are without excuse. For it is not those who hear the law who are righteous in God's sight, but it is those who obey the law who will be declared righteous.

The creation itself leaves these wrongdoers with no excuse. Although Gentiles may have never heard of the first commandment that we are to have no false gods, they nevertheless could come to this knowledge in a natural way. Since the creation of Adam and Eve, that is, before the coming of Christ or the giving of the Decalogue, human beings have had no excuse for their wrongdoing. Even without the "law" revealed first to Moses and fulfilled in Christ, human beings by nature can know right from wrong; hence, they can sin.[18]

This truth magnifies the greatness of Christ insofar as it makes humankind even more in need of His grace and forgiveness. If humankind could have no knowledge of right and wrong apart from revelation, then the majority of mankind would still be like little children whose mental incapacity prevents them from any moral wrongdoing whatsoever. But surely the universal message of sin, "all have sinned and fall short of the glory of God" (Rom. 3:23), and the universal good news of redemption, presuppose that human beings of the age of reason can discern right from wrong. Certainly, they cannot always do this perfectly. However, normally functioning people of the age of reason are responsible for knowing that certain grossly immoral acts are not to be done, e.g., idolatry, murder, adultery, and theft.

Patristic authors support this view and do not reject the usefulness of wisdom gleaned from pagan sources. The example of Augustine's stance towards "secular philosophy" may be instructive here. In *De Doctrina Christiana,* when treating the relationship of secular learning to sacred, Augustine recalls the Biblical precedent of the Jews stealing gold from the Egyptians. Just as the Jews took what was worth taking from the Egyptians, so Christians need not be opposed to the true, the good, and the beautiful no matter what their original source because anything true, good, and beautiful comes from the God of truth, goodness, and beauty.[19] Having experienced the aid of philosophy in his own conversion through reading Cicero's *Hortensius* and works of Platonic philosophy, Augustine believed that reason alone could discover moral truths also made known by revelation, and he himself sought to do this in his work *De Moribus Ecclesiae Catholicae.* One may object that other patristic authorities, particularly of the East, do not share Augustine's view. However, a similar case could be made with the Eastern Fathers, as well, by noting their adoption of Stoic and particularly neo-Platonic influences in both speculative and practical theology.

Secondly, theology does not determine all philosophical questions. The view that faith and philosophy are antagonistic competitors overlooks the fact that at least sometimes faith and philosophy are not competing in the same game. Engelhardt writes, "Christians are separated from others by their epistemology, their metaphysics, their understanding of history, their axiology, their appreciation of the sociology of knowledge and value, and the exemplars that direct their actions."[20] This passage makes it sound as if Christians had one view of these matters and their secular opponents the opposing view. Certainly, some philosophical perspectives on these matters are incompatible with Christianity—say, reductive materialism. However, there is a wide range of views that are compatible. With respect to these matters, among Christians, there is no single view that they themselves share. Consider, for instance, the views of epistemology advocated by various Christians. Bonaventure's Augustinian theory of divine illumination, Aquinas's theory of phantasms abstracted from the senses, and Alvin Plantinga's theory of properly constituted rational faculties offer very different epistemological accounts of how we come to know, but according to this account they are not respectively more or less Christian.[21] One could easily replace this example with one taken from metaphysics, history, or ethics. About a great many matters scientific, historical, and certainly philosophical, Christianity has no "single" program, solution, or answer. Needless to say, secular philosophy likewise cannot be understood as a single enterprise. "The" Christian view of epistemology, metaphysics, etc. cannot compete with "the" view of non-Christians insofar as Christians are divided among themselves and adopt, in whole or in part, various epistemological and metaphysical accounts.

Thirdly, theologies, indeed almost any expressions of the faith, almost inevitably presuppose philosophy, if only implicitly. Engelhardt, for example, seems to make use of what was originally a Stoic view of the passions as always morally suspect, a Neoplatonic account of "energies" of God, and a Platonic conception of the soul as divided into the intelligent, appetitive, and affective aspects.[22] Later, he employs the neo-Thomistic distinction between "direct" and "indirect" killing, a distinction whose relevance and parsing are not, at least not clearly, the subject of revelation but rather of philosophy. These philosophic elements are all derived, perhaps via patristic influence, but originally from what might be called "secular philosophers," that is, persons reasoning from premises available to believer and unbeliever alike. Although its influence may not be explicitly recognized, most theologians, including theologians opposed to what they take to be secular philosophy, adopt presuppositions, distinctions, outlooks, and arguments that can be traced to secular philosophy. One need not conclude that all such theologians are to that very extent in error.

Fourthly, Aquinas's view of the relationship of faith and reason seems to be vindicated insofar as secular philosophy has proved useful in removing objections to Christian morality. Secular philosophy has given reason to doubt a number of ethical theories such as emotivism, relativism, and consequentialism that, if true, would require rejection of Christian moral practice. Consider, for instance, secular philosophy's devastating critiques of consequentialism, a theory often invoked to support physician-assisted suicide. The critiques of consequentialism are legion; let us consider just one attack on this theory by a prominent secular philosopher. Bernard Williams has pointed out that consequentialism alienates the agent both from his own action and from a sense of community. In his essay "Utilitarianism: For and Against," Williams points out that on the consequentialist model of moral reasoning, individual aspirations, desires, and plans must all be offered for sacrifice on the altar of maximization. Human action becomes like a machine that produces a product labeled "best state of affairs" without regard for any other considerations. If one would bring about the most good as a medical technician in a remote village in Africa, one is morally obligated to do this and only this, regardless of personal preferences or inclinations. One may foster the personal relationships of marriage, family, and friendship, if and only if it leads to maximizing the good for all concerned. That an action results in your own mother, brother, or spouse dying in agony does not make any difference in the calculation of the best state of affairs. Williams's arguments against consequentialism have been widely influential in the secular philosophical community and have contributed to the conclusion of most ethicists that consequentialism must be rejected. One could cite philosophical critiques of relativism, emotivism, and other moral theories incompatible with Christianity. Certainly, these philosophies sometimes also reject the conclusions of Christian morality, but their critiques of anti-Christian morality may be useful and true nonetheless. Non-Christian philosophy can, particularly when practiced by the Christian, be used to remove objections to faith, as so many apologists from the scholarly Alvin Plantinga to the popular Fulton Sheen have made clear.

Fifth and finally, "secular" philosophy has often condemned the practice of suicide and by extension physician-assisted suicide. Some important contemporary ethicists do support physician-assisted suicide. Dworkin, Nagel, Nozick, Rawls, and Thomson, all of whom support physican-assisted suicide, together submitted an amici curiae "philosopher's brief" to the Supreme Court when it had before it two cases related to physician-assisted suicide. Perhaps a majority of the present members of the American Philosophical Association also support physician-assisted suicide, but a significant number of both theistic and atheistic philosophers do not. In fact, the history of philosophy provides many examples of prominent philosophers who rejected suicide. The ancient world clustered all sorts of "wisdom" under the rubric of "philosophy." Hence, philosophy in the ancient world was closely associated with medicine. The Hippocratic Oath provides an early statement that euthanasia is incompatible with the proper functioning of the activity of medicine. Plato in the *Phaedo* (62a–d) recounts Socrates arguing against self-chosen death. Of course, medieval philosophy from Augustine through Aquinas likewise condemned suicide as unnatural and an act incompatible with human flourishing.

A significant number of philosophers of the modern period also offer a basis for arguments against suicide. For example, Thomas Hobbes and John Locke both believed that one's right to liberty was for the sake of preserving one's life:[23] hence any use of liberty against one's own life would not have rational justification. Because all liberty rights arise from the right to life, one simply cannot have a liberty right to end one's life, for this would undermine the original source of the liberty right. If one may not sell oneself into slavery, which would be to waive one's liberty right, then one certainly may not waive the right to life by permitting one's death through physician-assisted suicide, for it is this right to life which is the source of all liberty rights. Famously, Immanuel Kant states in *Grundlegung zur Metaphysik der Sitten* that:

> [If a person] does away with himself in order to avoid a painful situation, he makes use of a person merely as a means to attaining a tolerable state of affairs till the end of life. Man however is not a thing—not something that may be used merely as a means; he must always in his actions be regarded as an end in himself.[24]

Even John Stuart Mill's *Utilitarianism,* at least insofar as it may be read as an advocacy of rule utilitarianism, could be used as an argument against physician-assisted suicide. Speaking of the rule prohibiting lying, Mill writes, "We feel that the violation, for a present advantage, of a rule of such transcendent expediency is not expedient."[25] If rules forbidding lying are of such expediency that they are practically exceptionless norms, a fortiori rules forbidding killing innocent persons would be rules of such expediency. If physician-assisted suicide leads to many unfortunate consequences—such as an undermining of respect for human life, an abuse of the health care system based on a crude cost-benefit analysis, and an open door to killing for reasons other than pain relief—then a rule absolutely forbidding physician-assisted suicide would be of the utmost expediency. Unaided reason can offer sound arguments that actually support a condemnation of physician-assisted suicide without any appeal to revelation.[26] If any one of the arguments alluded to above establishes the illegitimacy of physician assisted-suicide, Aquinas's contention about the relationship of faith to reason finds powerful support. And even if none of these arguments turns out to be good defense of the Christian prohibition of physician-assisted suicide, some philosophers have at least sought to provide numerous arguments explicitly, or at least implicitly, in favor of the Church's condemnation of physician-assisted suicide. To this extent, philosophy has proven a friend, albeit a weak friend, of the Christian faith.

Although Thomasma and Engelhardt disagree with one another about the permissibility of physician-assisted suicide, they agree in approaching the matter in a way that implicitly rejects the Thomistic conception of the relationship between faith and reason. According to the

Thomistic view, proper philosophical argument does not lead to an abandonment of what one knows by faith. Faith and reason cannot be opposed because they both approach the truth that comes ultimately from God, faith in a complete and perfect way and philosophy in an incomplete and imperfect way. Alleged conflicts between faith and philosophy are just that—alleged conflicts. In fact, "secular" philosophy—if any of the arguments of Plato, Locke, Hobbes, Kant, or Mill are correct—can actually bring one to know the truth about issues such as physician-assisted suicide, but it naturally cannot bring one to the fullness of truth that is available through revelation. The enemy of the Christian faith is not, then, per se philosophy, be it in its ancient, modern, or postmodern forms, but rather erroneous philosophy—ancient, modern, or postmodern. To be sure, that is not in short supply. However, those who follow the Truth incarnated in the person of Christ should not fear any truth revealed by any light, be it the light of science, the light of philosophy, or the light of human experience.

Even among those who ostensibly agree that no doctor should intentionally kill his or her patient, there is no small disagreement about handling situations at the end of life, particularly when a person is permanently unconscious. Is it intentional euthanasia to withdraw nutrition and hydration from a person in a persistent vegetative state? If withdrawal of nutrition and hydration is made, does this constitute, sometimes or always, intentional killing? An intervention by Pope John Paul II on these questions prompted considerable discussion, and the next chapter looks at certain aspects of this discussion.

Ten

PVS Patients and Pope John Paul II

This chapter focuses on the ethics of removing artificially administered nutrition and hydration (ANH) from patients in permanent coma, post-coma unresponsiveness, or what is commonly but somewhat pejoratively called persistent vegetative state (PVS). A PVS state may be permanent and irreversible, or it may be temporary. Although the case of Teri Schindler Schiavo brought this condition to national attention, these reflections do not deal with the specific details of her moral, legal, and familial situation. Rather, they will focus on five issues raised by responses to the 2004 address of Pope John Paul II to participants at a Rome conference entitled "Life-Sustaining Treatments and Vegetative State: Scientific Advances and Ethical Dilemmas." These issues include:

(1) What is the exact authority of this papal teaching?
(2) Does the allocution require ANH in all cases for PVS patients, in almost all cases, as a general ideal that may be often unrealized, or in some other sense?
(3) Does this papal allocution represent a rejection or overturning of the longstanding Catholic tradition of distinguishing ordinary from extraordinary means?

(4) Is human life valuable and worth preserving even if no higher brain function is possible?

(5) Does this allocution, despite its obvious motivation to forward a "culture of life," in fact undermine such a culture?

While I will not in this chapter come to definitive conclusions about these matters and certainly will not provide a comprehensive review of the literature, I do hope to provide an overview of the major issues that have arisen from this address so that readers can get some sense of the debate that has formed in response to the allocution.

The Authority of Pope John Paul II's Allocution

James Bretzke, SJ, begins his discussion of the pope's allocution with some useful guidelines for exegesis and proper interpretation of Magisterial texts, noting that the character, the frequency, and the manner of the teaching are all relevant in determining the proper interpretation of a Magisterial teaching. Though helpful in many ways, Bretzke's emphasis tends to be somewhat reductionary in its account of the obedience due to the papal Magisterium. Bretzke correctly indicates that this allocution did not claim infallibility and that any teaching that is not infallible is therefore fallible. By definition, there is no middle way. Yet the issue of infallibility does not settle the problem of what stance should be taken towards this papal teaching. Far from invoking a spirit of minimalism, the Second Vatican Council taught that "religious submission of mind and will must be shown in a special way to the authentic Magisterium of the Roman Pontiff, *even when he is not speaking ex cathedra;* that is, it must be shown in such a way that his supreme Magisterium is acknowledged with reverence, the judgments made by him are sincerely adhered to, according to his manifest mind and will."[1] In discussion of the allocution, Kevin O'Rourke, OP, mentions in passing various "reversals" of Church teaching,[2] but it remains very much a matter in dispute whether developments of doctrine on such topics as lending at interest and religious liberty are properly characterized as "reversals."[3] Even though it is not an exercise of extraordinary papal infallibility, the allocution is properly described as an act of the papal Magisterium.

Is ANH Required for PVS Patients?

Adopting a minority perspective, Bretzke believes that the pope did not in fact affirm that hydration and nutrition even by artificial means had to be provided to patients in a persistent vegetative state. Bretzke writes: "Only when both the *finis operis* and the *finis operantis* are taken together in a set of concrete circumstances can the moral meaning of the action be adequately evaluated."[4] Much hinges on what is meant by "adequately evaluated." If this phrase means that one cannot come to a complete evaluation of the situation morally, then it is unproblematic. If someone does something intrinsically evil, then one cannot come to a complete evaluation of the situation—including the agent's culpability and the degree of departure from the rule of charity—without knowledge of the concrete circumstances and intention as well as the action itself. But one can, simply from knowing the *finis operis,* sometimes also called the object of the human act, have adequate knowledge of whether that *finis operis* was morally permissible without knowledge of the further intentions (in the sense of motivations) and circumstances surrounding performance of the act. At least, that is the teaching of Pope John Paul II in *Veritatis Splendor:* "Consequently, without in the least denying the influence on morality exercised by circumstances and especially by intentions, the Church teaches that 'there exist acts which *per se* and in themselves, independently of circumstances, are always seriously wrong by reason of their object.'"[5] Applying this principle to the case at hand is made more complicated because removal of ANH is not per se evil as is say adultery or perjury unless it is performed with the intention of killing as an act of euthanasia by omission. One could remove ANH licitly, all agree, in cases in which a person can no longer assimilate the nutrients or in cases in which death is imminent and nutrition and hydration no longer benefit the patient. Bretzke views the removal of Schiavo's feeding tube as such a case. "Terri Schiavo's feeding tube could be morally removed [because] its removal was not intended to cause her death, but rather that the *finis operas* [sic]/*operantis* of the withdrawal of the ANH was the intended removal of the last artificial obstacle to the completion of the dying process."[6] Likewise, John C. Harvey asserts that such individuals in a PVS have a "fatal pathology" because "they die of starvation and dehydration if medical intervention is not made."[7]

Bretzke and Harvey's analysis does not seem to comport with the facts of the case. Schiavo was not in the dying process, at least as commonly understood. If provided with ANH, she would have continued to live. Her death was in no sense imminent, nor was her death directly caused by the injuries she sustained years earlier. Rather the cause of her death was dehydration. PVS is simply not a fatal pathology, for no fatal pathology allows its victim to live for years, in some cases, for up to thirty-five years.[8]

In an article defending the allocution, William E. May described his and his colleagues' experiences learning from those who care for PVS patients:

> We learned that individuals in this condition are *not* suffering from a fatal pathology, that they are in a relatively stable condition and are capable of living for some time so long as they receive food and hydration. We learned that at the beginning they are capable of swallowing, but that feeding them orally takes a great deal of time and that using tubes to feed them lightens the burdens of their caregivers. We also learned that the cost of feeding them is very reasonable, and that they do not have to be kept in expensive institutions but can be cared for at home if someone is there to provide care and who can be helped by visiting nurses, etc.[9]

Indeed, if the medical facts are as May describes, one could with equal justification say that healthy newborns suffer from a fatal pathology because they can only survive if provided nourishment.

Likewise, reading the papal statement as providing more leeway for removal of ANH from PVS patients, John C. Harvey interprets the allocution's phrase "proper finality" as the restoration of full function, which is impossible for PVS patients whose condition was caused by anoxia (though not for PVS patients whose condition was caused by drug over-dose). Thus, ANH would be required for PVS patients who could recover full function, but it would not be required for those who could not. For cases of permanent PVS—as opposed to simply persistent, but not per-manent, nonresponsiveness—removal is warranted because the proper finality of the medical treatment, the cure of the PVS, is impossible, mak-ing all treatments aimed at this goal futile.[10]

A difficulty with this reading of the allocution is that Pope John Paul II expressly denies that ANH is a "medical treatment" but rather as-serts that it constitutes ordinary care. Another difficulty is that the allocu-tion simply does not distinguish between these two conditions (permanent PVS caused by anoxia vs. potentially reversible PVS caused by drug over-dose). Thus, making use of this distinction to interpret the teaching could arguably be viewed more as eisegesis than exegesis: reading one's own view into the text rather than properly understanding what the author was attempting to convey.

Most interpreters have read the allocution as requiring ANH for all PVS patients so long as the ANH is achieving the goal of sustaining human life—its proper finality. They have faulted or praised the speech on this basis.[11]

Papal Allocution and Catholic Tradition

Among those who fault the allocution as too restrictive, many have seen a contradiction between the allocution and the Catholic tradition with re-spect to which means of preserving life are obligatory and which are not required. Most of them draw on the 1958 Gregorian doctoral dissertation of Daniel A. Cronin, "The Moral Law in Regard to the Ordinary and Extraordinary Means of Conserving Life."[12] Citing such venerable au-thorities as Vitoria (d. 1546), Soto (d. 1560), Sayrus (d. 1602), Banez (d. 1604), and Gury (d. 1866), they argue that this papal allocution is in contradiction with these earlier understandings of what would constitute extraordinary (and thus non-obligatory) means of preserving life.

The role of tradition remains an important one for Catholic ethics, yet tradition is not always used consistently. The tradition—especially the more recent tradition—is hardly uniform on the proper uses of ANH. As Lisa Cahill notes, "Over the past several years, different theologians, bishops and bishops' conferences have offered differing views about whether and when artificial nutrition should be considered an extraordinary or disproportionate means."[13] Indeed, none of the cited scholastic authors dealt with the question at hand—should ANH be provided for PVS patients and, if so, when?—so what they would say about this question is a matter of extrapolation from what they said about other matters.

In my view, there is indeed some tension between the allocution and the teaching of the scholastic authors. It is curious, however, that so many contemporary authors come to the defense of the scholastic tradition against the papacy when most if not all of these scholastic authors would endorse what Aquinas had to say about the relationship between the theologians and the Magisterium: "We ought to abide by the authority of the Church rather than by that of an Augustine or a Jerome or of any doctor whatever."[14] Likewise, many of these contemporary theologians endorse changing Church teaching on contraception, despite a much more ancient, widespread, and explicit condemnation of the practice in the Roman Catholic tradition.[15] Moreover, contemporary theologians have not criticized other (apparent) papal departures from the tradition such as Pope John Paul II's teaching on capital punishment.[16] These uses of tradition by some contemporary theologians do not seem entirely consistent.

Human Life as Intrinsic Good

Many critics of the papal allocution accuse the pope of a "vitalism," a virtual idolatry of human life. They hold that continued life in such a condition is not a great benefit,[17] indeed not a benefit at all. For example, Lisa Sowle Cahill writes, "Leaving the tubes in place cannot be simplistically equated with acting in her interests, since it could reasonably be argued that 15 or more years of existence in a 'vegetative' state neither serves human dignity nor presents a fate that most reasonable people would obviously prefer to death."[18]

All defenders of the allocation, as far as I can tell, hold that life always constitutes a benefit for the person. Criticizing Cahill, Jorge Garcia writes the following:

> I think it incoherent to deny that life is always a benefit to a human being and can discern no disservice to human dignity in preserving a human life, in which dignity inheres as such and irrespective of the blocking of many normal capacities. On the contrary to deem such a life as beneath preservation is to deny its inherent status. Whether many reasonable people would prefer death to a long life in PVS is morally irrelevant, since they may seek escape in death out of despair and incomprehension before the prospect of such a limited existence. Even reasonable people, of course, form some preferences from irrational parts of the self.[19]

The obvious importance of the question, whether human life is always valuable, as well as its anthropological implications for one's conception of the human person, was explored already in earlier chapters. However, any anthropology that even implicitly drives a dualistic wedge between the "biological life" or "vegetative life" and the "human" or "personal" life of the human being risks a dualism incompatible with a sound understanding of the human person. A frank discussion of this matter among philosophers and theologians in the Catholic tradition may clarify not only disputes about the papal allocution and the Schiavo case but also fundamental approaches to some of the most important questions of our time.

The Allocution and the Culture of Life

Finally, despite the pope's obvious intentions to the contrary, some writers criticize the papal allocution for undermining a culture of life and driving greater numbers of people towards direct euthanasia and physician-assisted suicide as a response to guidelines that are too restrictive.[20] I think it more likely that permitting removal of ANH for PVS patients in order to kill them will hasten the call for more expeditious forms of euthanasia and physician-assisted suicide. After all, it seems more compassionate to the patient and to those who watch the end of the patient's life to quickly and easily dispatch the PVS patient with a lethal injection rather than watch a slow deterioration over the course of five to thirteen days from dehydration.

Another factor that is more or less present in these debates is the discussion about what constitutes death. While some would say that a PVS patient is dead, the consensus of those working in the Catholic intellectual tradition appears to be that such patients are still living. After all, no one debates about providing nutrition and hydration for a corpse. Concerning "brain death," a lively discussion has arisen as to whether neurological criteria are appropriate for determining death. Despite widespread need for transplantable organs, relatively little discussion has taken place about donors whose hearts are not beating. The ethics of organ donation from those with non-beating hearts is the subject of the following chapter.

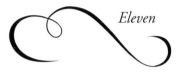

Eleven

Organ Donation after Cardiac Death

Organ donation after cardiac death (DCD), also known as non-heart-beating donation (NHBD) or non-heart-beating cadaveric donation (NHBCD), remains an issue of both ethical and practical interest, in part due to the increasing demand for viable organs. "The greatly enhanced technical ability to transplant organs has also led to an ever-increasing need for transplantable organs. The explosive growth in the demand for and the marginal increase in the supply of transplantable organs have together been characterized as an 'evolving national health care crisis.'"[1] In the United States, approximately 100,000 people are on organ-transplant waiting lists, but each year, only 10,000 to 20,000 patients receive organs.[2] DCD could narrow this gap. "Many patients in the intensive care unit will die of these very same neurological diagnoses but never satisfy criteria for brain stem death. It is by utilizing this new population of potential donors that NHBD (non-heart-beating donation) may substantially increase the organ donor pool."[3] It is estimated that DCD could increase the organ donor pool by twenty-five percent.[4] This possibility has generated considerable interest and pressure to facilitate DCD. A "federal mandate requires hospitals as of January 2007 to design policies and procedures for organ procurement in DCD to increase the rate of organ donation and recovery from decedents to 75 percent or greater."[5]

A second engine driving interest in DCD is the uncertainty as to whether brain death is truly death.[6] Before the use of neurological criteria to determine death, patients were declared dead using cardiopulmonary criteria (no heartbeat, no respiration), and organ transplantation could then follow. Today, most transplantation comes from brain-dead donors. Some organ donation, however, comes from cases where circulatory-respiratory criteria are used to determine death. However, if brain death is not truly death but rather the destruction of one extremely important— but not necessary—part of a human organism who continues to live in an irreversibly comatose and moribund state, then the use of neurological criteria to determine death should not be used. For purposes of determining death, we should use other criteria such as circulatory-respiratory functioning.[7]

DCD Controversies

Unfortunately, even DCD is ethically controversial. Presupposing the intrinsic dignity of every human being articulated earlier in this book, this chapter summarizes the current state of the debate and draws conclusions about transplantation from non-heart-beating donors. The ethical debate about DCD revolves around three questions.

First, can we resolve the potential conflicts of interest between providing the best care for the potential non-heart-beating donor and for the potential organ recipient? If donors are not given proper care because the medical team is more interested in harvesting their organs than in salvaging their lives, then this is not only an injustice to donors, but will also decrease the likelihood that others will wish to donate their organs when treated for serious injury or illness. Patients are less likely to sign up to donate their organs if there is a public perception that doctors provide less than suitable care for patients in order to harvest their organs.

Second, are ante-mortem interventions on the potential donor for the sake of obtaining his organs permissible? In ante-mortem interventions, the organs of the donor are treated prior to death in order to make them more suitable for donation. It is sometimes claimed that such ante-mortem interventions violate the principle that the human person should always be respected as an end and never used simply as a means. The human dignity of the donor must be respected, but an ethical concern arises that ante-mortem interventions might hasten the donor's death for the sake of the organ recipient. Others believe the contrary, that ante-mortem interventions on the potential donor—that is, the current patient—do not in fact use one person in order to aid another.

Third, when can we determine death by means of circulatory-respiratory criteria? In order to answer this question, it is necessary to determine exactly what "death" is and when it occurs. This third question is perhaps the most difficult because it involves consideration of various possible definitions of death, rival anatomical criteria for various definitions of death, and views about what clinical tests should determine that the criteria for death have been satisfied. A practical question connected with respective definitions of death is: How long will organs harvested by various means remain viable for transplantation?

In order to fruitfully consider these three questions, it is helpful to distinguish various kinds of non-heart-beating organ donation. The Maastricht categories have provided differentiation as follows: Category 1 is the "uncontrolled" scenario in which the patient is "dead on arrival"; Category 2 is "uncontrolled" unsuccessful resuscitation; Category 3 is "controlled" withdrawal of care in the critically ill; Category 4 is cardiac arrest after brain-stem death; and Category 5 is unexpected, "uncontrolled" cardiac arrest in a critically ill patient.[8] The difference between "controlled" DCD (Category 3) and "uncontrolled" DCD (Categories 1, 2, 4, and 5) will come into play as we answer the three sets of questions posed by our investigation of DCD.

The first set of questions concerns the debate about possible conflict of interest in DCD. Is there a conflict between providing the best possible care for the patient and looking out for the potential organ recipient? Is preparing the dying patient's organs for transplantation a conflict of interest with providing the best care possible for the dying patient? The potential conflict between proper care for the donor and care for the organ recipient is not at issue for Category 1 cases (uncontrolled DCD) because the donor has already died. So, the possible conflict can only arise in cases of controlled DCD.

As Zeiler and colleagues note, the Swedish Transplantation Act may provide a model for respecting the autonomy and medical needs of potential donors while also securing greater availability of organs for those in need.[9] In Sweden, the medical staff is strictly forbidden to discuss the potential donor's decision with the donor or the family during the course of treatment. If the medical staff does not know whether or not the patient has volunteered to be a donor, the medical staff does not have a motivation for treating patients in different ways based on their donor status. Only following declaration of death does the medical staff check the Registry for Organ Donation to determine whether the deceased patient had consented to donate his organs. This protocol defuses the potential conflict between the duty to care for the patient as an end in himself and the desire to care for other patients in need of organs. If discussion of donor status with medical staff prior to determination of death is strictly forbidden, the health-care team will have no incentive to change the course of care in one way or another in light of the patient's donor status—which remains unknown to the physicians until the patient's death is declared. Of course, there is still the possibility that the health-care team could give sub-par care to a potential donor, but this is true in all cases save where all donation is explicitly forbidden.

Ante-Mortem Interventions

What then of the second question about the permissibility of ante-mortem interventions on the donor solely for the sake of the potential recipient? In so-called Category 1 "uncontrolled" post-death scenarios, Swedish guidelines are not in play because the patient is dead and hence ante-mortem interventions are not possible. Ante-mortem interventions are possible only in cases of controlled DCD. In these cases, some may object to ante-mortem interventions because one person (the donor) is used simply as a means to help another person (the organ recipient). In ante-mortem interventions, the patient is not yet dead, but he is given medications for the benefit of another person, the future recipient of his organs. DCD is thus seen as dehumanizing to the organ donor. This dehumanization could even lead to the withdrawal of basic treatment needed to sustain the lives of those who are not in danger of death.[10] Valko argues further that seriously ill patients might encounter pressure to "pull the plug" and make themselves useful as a source of organ donation. This is a legitimate concern, especially in cultures in which the physically or mentally disabled, seriously diseased, and chronically dependent can be viewed as no longer possessing the equal, basic dignity of other human beings.

Unfortunately, some advocates of DCD portray the disabled in precisely these terms: "The decision to remove life supports from nonheart beating organ donors affirms a belief they are living in a state worse than death."[11] Such patients are viewed as "better off dead than alive with severe pain and discomfort."[12] These assertions are not sufficiently differentiated. It is true that severe pain, discomfort, and disability are undoubtedly evil, and that in order for these evils to exist, the being who endures them must be alive. But this does not mean that life itself is evil, nor does it mean that such patients are better off dead. Life is always a good because it is an intrinsic aspect of what it is to be a human being, and to be a human being is good. Knowing about a painful truth causes suffering, but it does not thereby cause human intelligence to become evil or something that one is better off not having. So, too, the evils that are made possible due to human life do not thereby render human life itself burdensome or not worth living.

May one licitly turn down treatment in order to aid another? "One unresolved question is whether altruistic patients who want to increase the chances that their deaths will produce usable organs may choose to alter the care provided in the last few hours of their lives."[13] But in standard practice, a competent patient always has the prerogative to refuse treatments as an expression of autonomy. So, if an altruistic and competent patient chooses to refuse or discontinue a treatment that in the patient's view is disproportional or not worthwhile in order to facilitate organ transplantation, it is difficult to see why this would be morally or legally problematic. Refusal or discontinuance of treatment used as a means to commit suicide would be ethically problematic, not just because of "bad publicity and the risks to organ procurement," but also and more fundamentally because such action would be intrinsically evil.[14] As Childress notes, "There are good moral and legal reasons to avoid the practice of killing patients, even with their consent, in order to provide transplantable organs."[15] However, refusal of treatment—not as a suicidal rejection of life but rather as a rejection of treatment considered more burdensome than beneficial—is not morally wrong. Likewise, refusal of treatment in order to benefit others may be seen as a nobler motive than refusing treatment simply because of the burdens the treatment imposes upon oneself.

Moreover, the removal of life support need not be motivated by a suicidal intent or a judgment that the patient's life is not worth living. Removal of any given treatment, including life support, may rest on the judgment that the treatment in question is no longer worthwhile, and this judgment in turn may follow from a variety of considerations including cost, the burden of the treatment, the diminishing returns the treatment is providing, or a free decision of a patient to forgo a treatment in order to conserve resources for others. In other words, the decision that a given *treatment* is not worthwhile need not presuppose that the *patient* is not worthwhile.[16]

In considering the ethical questions surrounding organ donation, the possible abuse of NHBD does not preclude legitimate use (*abusus non tollit usum*). Indeed, pushed to its logical extreme, the argument against NHBD that pressure to discontinue life support may be unfairly or immorally pushed on the seriously ill would suggest that it would always be wrong to discontinue life support on the understanding that any such allowance may lead to abuses. It is true that conflicts of interest in such cases provide one further motive to pressure someone towards death. Yet potential conflicts need not be actual conflicts of interest, and there may be many other motivations (such as children wanting an inheritance) that do not by themselves require extending care as long as possible.

Another proposed norm for governing non-heart-beating donation is articulated by the University of Pittsburgh Medical Center policy that "all interventions must be justified by their being effective in the care of the patient. No interventions are to be justified by their being effective in preserving a more usable transplant or in regulating the time of death."[17] In a similar manner, Peter Clark and Uday Deshmukh propose that "there must be no administration of anticoagulants or vasodilators (for example, heparin, phenotolamine) premortem."[18]

These policies, however, are surely too stringent. In other cases of transplantation, such as donating a single kidney with informed consent, the donor accepts risks in order to donate. An appeal to altruism has also been used to justify the use of treatments that may harm the organ donor for the sake of the organ recipient.[19] Altruism describes a person's willingness to risk or accept harm for the sake of helping others. Blood donors in a minor way and kidney and (partial) liver donors risk more serious harm and accept suffering for the sake of giving life to others. Steinberg argues that "we can at least evaluate the risk to a nonheart beating organ donor in the context of a society that permits a small risk of death and a more significant risk of morbidity in healthy living donors who otherwise might anticipate decades of good quality living. By this comparison, the risks of ante-mortem heparin are minimal and should be acceptable."[20] In the DCD case, the donor is taking no additional lethal risk because death is coming with certainty (given the decision to withdraw care), so ante-mortem interventions would seem even easier to justify than the widely accepted case of donating one kidney, in which case the donor is not doomed to die given the withdrawal of other care. As long as informed consent has been given, kidney donations do not violate the Kantian principle of respect because one is not making use of another person simply as a means because an autonomous donor has endorsed providing this generous gift of his kidney. Of course, there are limits beyond which abundant generosity ends and violations of proper self-love and self-regard begin. To risk one's well-being in giving a kidney is heroically generous; to kill oneself in order to provide organs for others violates the principle that no innocent person—including oneself—should be intentionally killed.

But perhaps on these grounds an objection can be lodged against ante-mortem interventions in DCD cases: one may not intentionally kill oneself nor even hasten one's death to aid another person. In uncontrolled cases of DCD, these issues are not relevant because the person cannot be revived. But in controlled cases, removal of life support need not be intentional killing. Indeed, when done ethically, such removal is based in recognition that a given treatment is more burdensome than beneficial, and therefore the life support may be removed. The judgment is not that the person's life is more burdensome than beneficial but rather that the given treatment is more burdensome than beneficial. So, assuming a lack of homicidal intent, removing life support in this manner is ethically acceptable. In other words, removal of life support, not to mention ante-mortem interventions, need not involve intentional killing. But do ante-mortem interventions on the potential donor hasten death? It does not appear that any of the typical ante-mortem interventions used in DCD cases, such as heparin, regitine, phentolamine, or cannulation, hasten death in potential NHB donors. However, many authors state that such interventions have risks, perhaps even lethal risks.[21]

Even if these interventions did risk hastening death in some cases, doing some action that has a possible or even certain evil side effect is ethically permissible if certain conditions are met. Double-effect reasoning, or the so-called principle of double effect, describes what conditions need to be met in order for an action with two (or more) effects, some good and some evil, to be justified. Double-effect reasoning can justify ante-mortem interventions in DCD cases. The first condition to consider is that such interventions are not intrinsically evil, even if they risk death, for risking death for a serious reason is itself permissible. Secondly, the foreseen potential evil that the patient's death may be hastened is not a means to the end because it is not the donor's hastened death that makes the organs more suitable for transplantation. Third, the foreseen potential evil is not necessarily intended because the doctor is presumably not aiming, as a means or as an end, to bring about death through the preparation of the donor's organs prior to death. Finally, there is a proportionately serious reason for allowing the evil effect, namely saving another person's life.

On the other hand, some authors question whether double-effect reasoning can indeed justify ante-mortem interventions. Quoting Beauchamp and Childress with approval, Steinberg views the problem, in part, to be the fact that "almost anything can be foreseen as a side effect rather than intended as a means."[22] According to this view, double effect is a kind of ethical double-think. But this kind of use of double-effect reasoning is really an abuse, and as such is not an objection to double-effect reasoning per se. It is simply not the case that almost anything can be foreseen as a side effect rather than intended as a means. Even according to the most "narrow" accounts of intention, if an effect is chosen so as to bring about another effect, then that effect is an intentionally chosen means, and it is therefore intended regardless of narrative rationalizations of the agent. In Letter 7 of the *Provincial Letters,* Blaise Pascal critiqued what he viewed as perniciously lax Jesuitical exhortations to direct one's intention in one way rather than another so as to accomplish "ethically" what was in fact morally wrong.[23] Again citing Beauchamp and Childress with approval, Steinberg lodges a similar objection, that "the principle of double-effect can be manipulated because the notion of what is intended is both malleable and subject to the whims of human consciousness. The same act may be permissible or impermissible depending on what enters a physician's consciousness."[24] According to this view, then, double-effect reasoning leads to a relativistic subjectivism.

Steinberg's objection is undifferentiated. If an aspect of the act is literally unknown to the agent, if it does not enter into the agent's consciousness at all, then that aspect of what is done is performed in ignorance. If the ignorance involved is inculpable, then the agent is not morally responsible for the effect. The act, as chosen, is not defined by the unknown effect. If the ignorance is culpable, then the agent is morally responsible for whatever bad effects follow from the act. Is what is intended "malleable" in the sense that one can choose some act, or the effect of some act, as a means and, by mere mental focus, make the act permissible? No, whatever is chosen as a means or as an end in itself is intended, whatever story one tells oneself, whatever one's mental focus, whatever one's state of emotion. Indeed, what one intends is not infinitely plastic but rather corresponds to the actual means and actual ends chosen as a product of one's practical reasoning.

Zeiler and colleagues, also, argue that the patient should be treated only for his or her own sake and that therefore the use of anticoagulants and other drugs for the sake of the person receiving the donation is prohibited.[25] Their rationale is that this provision is required in order to maintain public trust in the health-care system. A lack of public trust in health-care providers drives down the number of willing organ donors.

However, if a person gives truly informed consent for such treatments, especially when such consent is legally documented in a living will and orally confirmed prior to ante-mortem interventions, it is difficult to see why public trust in the health-care system would be undermined. After all, when a healthy person donates a kidney, consent is given for medical procedures to be performed on the donor solely for the medical good of the recipient, yet this is not viewed as problematic. Indeed, DCD is even less problematic insofar as the donor, who is already in the process of dying, has much less to risk and much less to lose than the healthy donor. In DCD, death is not risked (since it is a certainty anyway). In healthy organ donation, death is risked.

Let us posit for the sake of argument that the prior arguments addressing the permissibility of ante-mortem interventions are mistaken. Imagine that there were conclusive evidence that the typical ante-mortem interventions hastened death, that we did not already accept medical interventions on one patient solely for the sake of another (kidney transplant), and that double-effect reasoning could not justify such interventions. Would DCD thereby be impermissible? No, because ante-mortem interventions are not necessary for DCD, so those who object to their use can forgo them, though the viability of their organs will thereby also be reduced.

Determination of Death

The third and most difficult set of questions about DCD surrounds the determination of death. I will presuppose but not defend in this chapter the "dead donor rule," that vital organs may not be taken from a donor prior to death. Therefore, we may not take vital organs from a living person, if doing so amounts to murder. In DCD, then, the person must be truly dead before his organs can be removed, and it becomes important to determine when death occurs.[26] It is important to distinguish (1) the definition or concept of death, (2) the anatomical criteria that instantiate the definition, and (3) the clinical signs or tests that determine whether the anatomical criteria have been met.[27] I am not going to discuss the third aspect, as this type of analysis should be left to medical professionals. Rather, I will focus on the concept or definition of death and the anatomical criteria that instantiate this definition.

Definitions of Death

What is the definition or concept of death? Death can be defined socio-
logically, psychologically, and biologically.[28] The sociological definition of
death is simply whatever a community consensus determines. This definition can vary widely from community to community. Within a multi-
cultural community, one and the same being could be considered alive by
some subgroups of the community and dead by other subgroups of the
community. This nominal definition of death is deeply relativistic, and
insofar as moral relativism is problematic as a basis for making sound
moral decisions, this definition of death should be rejected.

A second definition of death is a psychological definition specific to
human persons, who are equated with functioning minds. According to
this definition, a human person can die, but the human being/body formerly related to that mind can continue to live. This definition, too, is
problematic, in part because it rests on a erroneous body-self dualism,
and, as with the sociological definition of death, I will merely register my
disagreement before turning to the biological definition of death.[29]

The biological definition of death is the irreversible cessation of the
integrated functioning of the organism as a whole. Unlike the psychological definition of death, this definition is not species-specific but holds
true for organisms as genetically simple as plant parasites or as genetically
complex as marbled lungfish. Unlike the sociological definition, the
meaning or intension of the biological definition is not culturally relative,
even if the extension or connotation of the biological definition might be
subject to dispute in borderline cases.

Anatomical Criteria

If we adopt the biological definition of death, what are the anatomical
criteria that instantiate this definition? The Uniform Determination of
Death Act accepts "cardiac death" or "brain death" as fulfilling the biological definition of death. "An individual who has sustained either (1)
irreversible cessation of circulatory and respiratory functions, or (2) irreversible cessation of all functions of the entire brain, including the brain

stem, is dead."[30] If we also accept those criteria, how should we understand "irreversible cessation" here? There are at least three interpretations of irreversible cessation: First, irreversible cessation could mean that it is not logically possible to reverse the loss of function. Second, it could mean an inability to autoreverse, to self-resuscitate, combined with the ethical impermissibility of others attempting to reverse function. Finally, irreversible function could be interpreted to mean that there is a loss of function even in spite of technological intervention, regardless of whether or not it is ethically permissible to intervene. Let us consider each interpretation in turn.

Taking the first interpretation, we could interpret "irreversible cessation" to mean that a person is dead only if it is not logically possible to reverse loss of function. According to this interpretation, human beings are dead when the very idea of bringing them back to life would be like constructing a square circle. Irreversible in this sense means logically impossible under any circumstances whatsoever. I am aware of no philosophical argument for the conclusion that it is logically impossible to raise the dead. Intuitively, a square circle and the dead coming back to life are very different, for one cannot even imagine a square circle, but one can easily imagine a person rising from the dead. Interpreting irreversible cessation in the definition of death to mean "logically impossible to reverse function" is also deeply problematic in terms of organ donation. Even those who have long ceased any vital function—John F. Kennedy, John Milton, or John the Baptist—would not be counted as dead because the restoration of their vital functions is imaginable and therefore logically possible.

Moreover, the first interpretation, defining "irreversibility" as logical impossibility, is incompatible with many religious beliefs, including accounts of raising the dead in the Buddhist, Christian, Muslim, and Jewish faiths. For example, Christian Scripture describes numerous cases of Jesus raising the dead (e.g., Lazarus, the daughter of Jairus, and the widow's son). These accounts, and similar accounts in other religious traditions, imply both that certain human beings were really dead and that in the actual world such people did not have "irreversible cessation" of function in a logically impossible sense. What is logically impossible can happen in no world and anything that did happen in the actual world is a fortiori logically possible.[31] So, no orthdodox Christian, Buddhist, Muslim, or Jew can accept this understanding of irreversible cessation.

The second interpretation defines "irreversible cessation" as the inability to autoreverse even though the person could be revived through morally impermissible medical intervention. DuBois understands "irreversibility" to mean ethically irreversible, such that it would be morally and legally impermissible to revive the person even though the empirical possibility of reviving the person remains open.[32] A human being has died when their circulatory functions cannot autoreverse and it would be wrong for a medical team to attempt to restart cardiocirculatory functions, such as when a DNR (Do Not Resuscitate) order is in place.

This view is problematic, for it implies that many people—hundreds and perhaps thousands a year—have died and come back to life through human intervention, albeit ethically impermissible human intervention. It is more accurate to say that persons with the inability to autoreverse their lack of heartbeat are dying, but that they are not dead yet. Otherwise, we are forced to say that people can "die" numerous times, and that people are often raised from the dead by simple CPR. To this objection, DuBois responds:

> Some may find this concept of irreversibility problematic, because it implies that death is sometimes reversible. Yet the idea of a reversible state of death is not only consistent with certain theological concepts (such as the resurrection of the dead) and controversial reports of near death experiences by those determined to be clinically dead, but it is simply logical. In order to determine that a body is permanently in a certain state (for example, the state of being frozen, being comatose, or being dead), one must first be able to verify that the person is in the state. That is, the concept of being in a given state is necessarily prior to the concept of being irreversibly in that state.[33]

What is meant here by the word "prior"? As Aristotle pointed out in the *Categories,* book 12, one thing can be prior or primary to another in various ways: (1) by order of time, as Socrates was prior to Descartes; (2) if one thing requires the existence of another, but not the converse, as getting a tan requires skin, but having skin does not require getting a tan;

(3) in some particular order, as "alligator" is prior to "cat" in alphabetical order; or (4) by declaring one thing as more important, honorable, or better than another, as the prime minister is more important than auxiliary ministers.[34] DuBois is correct that the concept of being in a given state is necessarily prior (Aristotle's case 2, not his case 1) to the concept of being irreversibly in that state in that you must, in the metaphysical order, be dead as a necessary condition to being irreversibly dead. But metaphysical priority does not imply chronological priority. For example, a wife losing her husband to death is prior to her becoming a widow metaphysically because losing her husband is the cause of her becoming a widow. However, her husband's death is not prior chronologically to her becoming a widow because she becomes a widow at the very moment her husband dies. So, not all that is metaphysically prior is also chronologically prior. Dubois's argument is logically invalid because it plays on the metaphysical and chronological ambiguity of the word "prior."

There are other difficulties with interpreting "irreversibility" in the definition of death to mean ethically unacceptable to reverse. "The issue is not whether there are good reasons not to resuscitate a person," as Verheijde, Rady, and McGregor point out, "but whether the person is truly dead."[35] In Alexander Capron's words, "Irreversibility must mean more than simply 'we choose not to reverse, although we might have succeeded.'"[36]

This leads us to the third interpretation of irreversibility, namely the loss of function even with technological intervention. According to this view, a person has died when their life functions have irreversibly ceased, regardless of the life-support techniques used. A person is dead when vital functions cannot be restored despite maximal medical intervention. Of the views considered, this would seem by process of elimination to be the most reasonable one.

One objection raised against this view is that the transplantation of heart, lungs, or other vital organs indicates that function of heart or lungs has not been irreversibly lost.[37] If the heart and lungs are able to function, then there has not been an irreversible loss of function of the heart or lungs, so death has not taken place. On the other hand, if the vital organs cannot function, then transplantation is not medically useful for the organ recipient.

What is at issue, however, is whether a patient has lost cardiorespiratory function as a whole, not whether the heart or lungs no longer work in another patient. If a guillotine is used to kill a person, and the head thrown into a vat of acid, that person is uncontroversially dead, but the organs of that person may very well be viable for transplantation into another person. In a more realistic example, heart disease may bring about the death of the donor and render the heart unsuitable for transplantation, but the donor's lungs may still remain viable for transplantation. In other cases, lung cancer causes death and renders the lungs useless for transplantation, yet the heart may still function well in another person. What is at issue in determining death is whether there is irreversible loss of cardiopulmonary function in a given patient, not whether the lungs themselves or the heart itself is incapable of function in another person.

Application to DCD

When does irreversible loss of cardiopulmonary or, in D. Alan Shewmon's terms, circulatory-respiratory function happen? There is no agreement about the timeline of determination of death by cardiopulmonary criteria. In many ICUs, patients are certified dead after less than two minutes of asystole. The Pittsburgh protocol for DCD draws the line at two minutes, the Institute of Medicine at five minutes, and the Maastricht protocol at ten minutes. Shewmon, the foremost critic of brain death, holds that in typical cases, the "point of no return" is twenty to thirty minutes after loss of circulation.[38] Shewmon's standard is the most demanding of which I am aware.

In cases of uncontrolled DCD, it would seem that death has already taken place because restoration of function has failed. So, in such cases, it would not seem to violate the dead-donor rule to remove organs. In most cases, the family cannot be notified prior to donation, but if the person had already consented to becoming a donor, then it is not ethically necessary to also secure the family's consent. One consideration is whether acceding to the donor's consent without the express authorization of the family might, over time, drive down the number of potential donors; another is whether going ahead with donation without the authorization of the family might subject the hospital to legal liability. Whether or not these unfortunate results would come to pass is an important question, but it is not relevant in terms of assessing the ethics of uncontrolled DCD in itself and in circumstances which may vary widely.

In some very rare cases, however, uncontrolled DCD would be ethically unacceptable, at least in those situations where prior resuscitation attempts have been made. The so-called Lazarus syndrome, also sometimes called the Lazarus phenomenon, describes rare cases in which the patient's heart spontaneously resumes beating after CPR to restore life was attempted and was thought to have failed.[39] In cases of failed resuscitation, the possibility of the Lazarus syndrome would lead to the ethical conclusion that uncontrolled DCD is morally impermissible on account of the risk (albeit very small) that the patient could recover, even fully recover, after apparently failed CPR attempts. Removing vital organs in cases where the Lazarus effect would otherwise have taken place is killing the patient to aid another person. However, there is no reported case of the Lazarus phenomenon having taken place after two minutes unless there had been prior attempts at resuscitation.[40] Thus uncontrolled DCD is permissible after two minutes if there were no prior resuscitation attempts. Cases in which resuscitation was attempted and apparently failed should therefore be treated as cases of controlled DCD, as I will discuss next.

In controlled DCD, when does irreversible loss of function, even with technological intervention, occur? If we adopt the most demanding standard, so as to have the maximum assurance that we are not violating the dead-donor rule, the "point of no return" is probably some twenty to thirty minutes following final loss of cardiopulmonary function. Exceptions to this general rule would include very young patients, victims of hypothermia, and people suffering from drug overdose. In standard cases, however, the patient is considered to have died after twenty or thirty minutes according to even the most demanding standard.

The advantage of adopting the most demanding standard is that we have the maximum assurance that we are not killing one person to save another compatible with organ retrieval. In addition to the ethical certainty of this view, an additional advantage is that it lessens the likelihood that the public will perceive transplantation as unethical—as intentionally killing one person to save another—a perception that can drive down the number of people willing to be donors and thus further exacerbate the organ shortage.

The difficulty with adopting the most demanding standard is that after twenty or thirty minutes of noncirculation of oxygenated blood, organs begin to deteriorate, making successful organ transplant less likely, if not impossible. Hence there arises the DCD dilemma: either take organs sooner, in which case we possibly violate the dead-donor rule and risk undermining public perceptions of organ donation, or observe the most demanding standard, in which case the organs will be less or even no longer viable.

A possible response involves escaping one horn of the dilemma, that the demanding standard renders organs useless for transplantation. Let us assume the donor has consented to both donation of his organs and removal of life support. After making a judgment that a given life-supporting treatment is more burdensome than beneficial, and after removing this treatment from the patient, the health-care team should wait until the heart cannot autoreverse, which is after two minutes of asystole in typical cases. How long must one wait to be sure that autoreversal is impossible? It does not really matter. If the demanding standard is correct, even if the heart did restart on its own after twenty to thirty minutes, restoration of integrated functioning would still not be possible, even with human intervention.

In a typical case of controlled DCD, what would happen? After two minutes, the team would administer ante-mortem drugs to better preserve the organs. (This stage could also be done prior to removing life support with informed consent.) Once the heart can no longer autoreverse, the medical team does everything necessary for removal of the organs—short of actually removing them—which, in this context, does not intentionally cause or even hasten death.[41] Following actual death, twenty to thirty minutes after the last heartbeat, the vital organs are removed from the body.

Is twenty or thirty minutes too long to wait for viable organs? The brain is the most sensitive of all the organs to oxygen deprivation, but of course, brain transplants are not currently possible. Therefore, the fact that the brain is non-functional after ten minutes without oxygenated blood is irrelevant for DCD (though perhaps very relevant if one determines death by neurological criteria). Livers and kidneys are the organs most often recovered from DCD.[42] Fortunately, livers and kidneys can be donated "up to forty minutes after cessation of heartbeat. (Kidneys and livers are more resilient to oxygen deprivation than other organs.)"[43] What about the lungs? "The gas exchange system of the lungs can tolerate one hour of warm ischemia after circulatory arrest without significant loss of functional capacity."[44] It may even be possible, but less promising, to transplant hearts while respecting the demanding standard, at least in its twenty-minute rather than thirty-minute form. "Recently the Papworth hospital group described the first case of functional recovery in a human deceased donor heart following in-vivo perfusion of the coronary circulation with normothermic blood using an extracorporeal circuit. After twenty-three minutes of warm ischemia the asystolic heart was perfused and reverted into sinus rhythm."[45] Livers, kidneys, lungs, and perhaps even hearts can be retrieved in cases of DCD, opening the door to more organ donation as well as an alternative to determining death by neurological criteria.

If kidneys, livers, lungs, and perhaps even hearts are all still viable after thirty minutes of asystole, then is not the patient really still alive? No, for as I mentioned earlier, the fact that an organ or even many organs may function well in a recipient's body does not mean that the donor did not die prior to removal of organs. Life requires the integrated functioning of the organism as a whole, not merely the functioning of various organs taken individually outside the context of the whole. Imagine a special disintegrating machine that destroyed every cell in the human body but the liver, lungs, heart, and kidneys. Such a disintegrated human being is obviously dead, but these organs are nevertheless viable. Life is not constituted by having various organs with the potentiality of participating in an integrally functioning organism but rather by being an organism with integrally functioning organs.

Conclusion

Three main ethical questions arise from DCD, and this chapter attempts to treat all three questions: whether the interests of the patient as donor and the potential organ recipient necessarily conflict, whether the use of ante-mortem drugs to facilitate organ transplantation are acceptable, and how to apply the dead-donor rule making use of cardiocirculatory criteria in cases of organ donation. Although practical hurdles remain to making organ transplantation more common—among them low donor rates—and although medical challenges remain to the successful transplantation of organs in some cases, the ethical issues surrounding DCD need not constrain those seeking to give life even in death.

But what should take place if a particular doctor does not believe that cardiocirculatory criteria constitute death? What if a person is declared brain dead, but a particular physician rejects neurological criteria for determining death? Should that physician be forced to transplant organs from a patient whom the doctor believes is still alive? Controversies over conscience usually revolve around issues at the beginning of life, but similar controversies can arise at the end of life, too. How should we handle cases where a patient's autonomy and a physician's conscience come into conflict? What rights, if any, do doctors, nurses, and other health care professionals have to refuse to do activities that in conscience they regard as immoral? It is to these questions of conscience to which we now turn.

Twelve

Conscience Protection and the Incompatibility Thesis

An operating-room nurse arrives at her weekend call shift. It is morning at Mount Sinai Hospital in New York City, and Cathy De-Carlo comes to her assignment desk just as she has countless times in her five years at the hospital. But this morning is different. Cathy is assigned to circulate in a room where a twenty-two-week "D&E" dismemberment abortion will be performed on a live baby. Cathy promptly calls for clarification, noting that the hospital has known her religious objection in writing based on her Catholic faith since the day she was hired. The pregnant mother is diagnosed with pre-eclampsia, but the hospital did not designate the case as requiring immediate surgery, and the patient is not on magnesium therapy. The patient later presents in the operating room in a stable condition with blood pressure that is not near crisis level. Cathy's supervisor, who is willing to participate in such procedures, is available to assist. And Mount Sinai, one of the top-ranked medical centers in the United States, receives hundreds of millions of federal health dollars every year, which require the hospital not to discriminate against employees who choose not to assist abortions if it would violate their religious beliefs. Yet despite Cathy's tearful pleas, her supervisors tell her she must immediately assist in the late-term abortion or she will be charged with insubordination and patient abandonment, threatening her job and her nursing license.[1]

Much is at stake in the debate about conscience, as the true story from Casey Mattox and Matthew S. Bowman makes clear. The dignity of persons, both as agents and as receivers of the action of other agents, is at stake. The contemporary debate has only intensified as those on all sides of the conscience debate hope to codify their views in law.

What is conscience? Although conscience is sometimes portrayed as a feeling or instinct, conscience is better understood as an agent's best reasoned judgment of whether or not to perform an action, reasoning which should be informed by careful consideration of moral truth and relevant circumstances. For Catholics, conscience should also be informed by prayer and the teachings of the Church. An action does not become morally right simply because it is done in accordance with conscience. Considered objectively as an action, to torture and murder an innocent person is always wrong. If someone's conscience compels him to torture and murder another person, it is difficult to avoid the conclusion that such an agent has voluntarily suppressed knowledge that he can and ought to know. Voluntary ignorance does not excuse an action that is morally wrong. Such a voluntarily ignorant agent is therefore guilty both of not properly informing his conscience and of harming and killing a person, the negative consequence that follows directly from his lack of due care in acting. An agent always has a moral obligation to obey his or her conscience, and a person always has a moral obligation to properly inform his or her conscience.

The prima facie case for respecting the consciences of others (including the right of others to refrain from activities that they regard as immoral) rests on basic principles that are widely shared. Prima facie, it is wrong to force another person to do anything, for in doing so, one makes the other person into simply a means to achieve one's own plans, as if that person were a tool or a slave. None of us want someone to force us to act against our consciences, so we should accord the same respect to others. Ceteris paribus, forcing someone to act against his or her conscience is not treating the person in accordance with respect for the dignity of that person.

There is a prima facie obligation to refrain from forcing others to violate their consciences. There are limits, however, to the actions that should be legally permitted in the public sphere, even if justified by conscience. For example, someone with a badly formed, erroneous conscience may think that he is justified in harming others because of their race. Those responsible for public order and safety may licitly punish such a person for his crimes, even though such crimes were undertaken at the behest of (erroneous) conscience. One of the most important questions now debated in bioethics is whether a physician who conscientiously refuses to perform an abortion or to provide contraception deserves respect for her conscience or ought to be punished, professionally or legally, for refusing to perform the actions requested of her position.

Mark R. Wicclair's essay "Is Conscientious Objection Incompatible with a Physician's Professional Obligations?" should be required reading for everyone involved in this discussion. Wicclair critiques the "incompatibility thesis," namely the view that, "anyone who is not willing to provide legally and professionally permitted medical services should choose another profession."[2] The first thing to remember about the incompatibility thesis is that it is a thesis, a proposition that is far from self-evident and needs a justification. Wicclair considers a wide array of different arguments for this conclusion, and he then concludes that each argument fails.

Consequentialist arguments hold that the incompatibility thesis is justified because it leads to overall greater well-being, especially for women seeking abortion and contraception. But, Wicclair points out, if likely overall consequences guide our decision making, then it is still far from clear that the incompatibility thesis is justified, especially if "well-being" includes the moral integrity of health care professionals and if other means are available to secure the desired services.[3]

This argument against the incompatibility thesis is strengthened by several considerations Wicclair does not mention. Vast numbers of people oppose abortion and believe it to be seriously wrong at least in most cases.

If performance of abortion is made a mandatory part of the medical profession, a great many doctors will be forced to step down from the practice of medicine, and a great number of talented young people will decide not to enter the profession.[4] As J.W. Gerrard notes, "The pragmatic reason [the incompatibility thesis fails] is that professions may have problems recruiting and retaining talented members in certain specialties if they do not find a way to accommodate divergent views."[5] Because, on average, more women than men are pro-life, as well as more Latinos than non-Latinos, and more people of faith than atheists, the self-selection against the practice of medicine would work against diversity among medical personnel. A similar point can be made about pro-life hospitals, many of which will shut down before being forced to perform abortions. "615 Catholic hospitals account for 12.5% of community hospitals in the United States, and over 15.5% of all U.S. hospital admissions."[6] To shut down these health care facilities will increase the cost of health care and put thousands of lives at risk. Those who care about women's health should consider not just the women who want abortions, but also the women, men, and children who have a wide variety of health care needs and who are endangered by forcing pro-life physicians and institutions out of medical practice.

If willingness to perform abortions is made a mandatory part of becoming a doctor, then a significant number of people who believe that abortion is the unjust intentional killing of an innocent person may join the medical profession anyway. This development would weaken the medical profession because these medical personnel who are willing to violate their consciences about such an important matter will probably be more likely to violate their consciences about other matters (such as falsifying insurance forms, lying to patients, or otherwise acting against what they take to be ethical behavior). This would harm the entire medical field. The practice of medicine would be further damaged by the public perception that physicians, not just as a group, but each individual physician, engage in practices that the majority of Americans find ethically problematic. This damages the prestige of the profession and undermines the trust that ought to exist between doctors and patients. These considerations suggest that the appeal to its consequences does not justify the incompatibility thesis.

Another possible justification of the incompatibility thesis is that physicians have a professional obligation to consider first and foremost the well-being of their patients. The professional obligations of physicians are characterized in different ways. One view "specifies the end of medicine as healing and . . . characterizes the physician-patient relationship as one between a professional committed to healing and a vulnerable patient who is ill and seeks help from the professional."[7] But the conscientious objector can reasonably claim that abortion is not an act of healing because pregnancy is not a disease and killing is not a healing act. Furthermore, as Wicclair points out, a physician can be committed to healing but decline to perform procedures that are sometimes used to heal others. Some doctors focus on one kind of specialty (i.e., dermatology), so they simply do not offer other kinds of treatments (i.e., hernia operations). They may decline to provide certain procedures simply because they prefer some kinds of treatments over others. If such demurrals to provide treatments are already permitted for reasons of mere preference, then how much more should demurrals be permitted for ethical reasons?

Perhaps the incompatibility thesis is justified because the physician has an obligation to place the interests of patients before the physician's own interests. However, as Wicclair argues, this duty is not absolute. Clearly, the physician should sometimes put the interests of the patient before his or her own. In the midst of performing a surgery, the doctor should not leave to play a round of golf. However, the duty to prioritize the interests of patients is not absolute. Doctors need not make house calls, cancel vacations, charge less or nothing at all, or schedule night time appointments to accommodate patients' schedules, although all of these actions may be in the interests of patients. Wicclair writes, "Any reasonable criterion would have to distinguish among interests according to their importance or significance and moral weight; and a physician's interest in moral integrity is a very important interest that has substantial moral weight."[8]

Another justification for the compatibility thesis rests on reciprocal justice. "Physicians enjoy certain rights, privileges, and benefits as professionals," writes Wicclair. "These include a monopoly to provide certain services, self-regulation, subsidized education and training, and government support for research."[9] In virtue of these privileges, they must provide requested services even if it violates their consciences. Wicclair argues that considerations of reciprocal justice also fail to ground the compatibility thesis.

> It is arguable that a requirement to provide services even when a pro-fessional has a conscience-based objection to doing so is no more rea-sonable than a requirement that physicians treat patients no matter how high the risk of death due to epidemics or bioterrorism. It is also arguable that more reasonable reciprocity-based requirements would set limits to risks and would permit conscientious objection with procedural requirements to protect patients, such as advance notifi-cation and referral. In any event, the reciprocal justice account fails to provide an unequivocal basis for the incompatibility thesis.[10]

We can accept that reciprocal justice entails that physicians have certain obligations to society and its ill members without holding that doctors should be forced to perform or to refer for abortion.

Another attempt to justify the incompatibility thesis is the promise model. According to this view, a person entering a particular medical spe-cialty has made a promise to future patients to provide the services that are typical and normal for the specialty. "In other words, individuals have a choice: become a member of a medical specialty or subspecialty and promise to provide the corresponding normal range of services, or, if pro-viding any of those services violates one's ethical and/or religious beliefs, select another medical specialty or subspecialty or another profession (i.e., one that is compatible with the individual's ethical and/or religious beliefs)."[11]

This justification, too, fails to provide unequivocal support for the incompatibility thesis. "Performing colonoscopies is a 'normal' or stan-dard procedure within gastroenterology, but not all gastroenterologists perform colonoscopies; and delivering babies is a 'normal' or standard practice within obstetrics/gynecology, but not all obstetrician/gynecolo-gists deliver babies. In neither case does a physician's failure to provide the service at issue constitute the breaking of a promise made upon entering her respective subspecialty."[12] There are, of course, certain "core" services that various specialties provide, such as performing pelvic examinations in gynecology. However, in a descriptive sense, it is implausible to claim that performing abortions is an essential element of being a gynecologist; thousands of gynecologists have never and will never perform abortions. To claim that it is essential, in an evaluative sense, is to beg the question. It is also implausible in the extreme to hold that all OB-GYNs have promised to perform abortions simply in virtue of becoming OB-GYNs, and if no promise has been made, then there is no promise to obligate. In sum, Wicclair's article provides a telling critique of the case against conscience rights for health care workers.

Cases raised by Dan Brock challenge the view presented by Wicclair.[13] In one example, Doctor A has deeply held racist beliefs and so refuses to treat persons of color who come into his practice. In another, Doctor B becomes a Jehovah's Witness and refuses to perform blood transfusions, even at the cost of a patient's life.[14] Brock holds that Doctor B should be told, "Transfusing patients when that is medically indicated is a central part of your role and responsibilities as an emergency physician. You freely chose that role knowing that this responsibility is an important part of it. If after doing so you have now adopted religious beliefs which prohibit you from carrying out this responsibility without violating your personal beliefs and moral integrity, then you must leave that role and the hospital would be justified in firing you if you do not."[15] Or, to change the case slightly, in the case of a gynecologist, the choice would be "perform the abortion or find a new job." Are the Doctor A and Doctor B examples similar to conscientious objection to abortion or contraception?

Doctor A's case is not analogous because it has to do with refusal to treat a certain kind of *person,* not a refusal to perform *certain kinds of procedures* for any kind of person. Discrimination against persons is significantly morally different than discrimination against particular kinds of actions. Nor is the case of Doctor B similar to conscientious objection to abortion and contraception. Aside from abortion to save the life of the mother (which does not actually qualify as abortion when abortion is properly defined as the intentional killing of the human fetus as a means or as an end in itself, and therefore not necessary to save the life of the mother),[16] one difference between the cases is that denial of transfusion leads to the death of the patient, but a denial of abortion does not lead to the death of either the patient who is the mother or the patient who is the unborn human being. Likewise, not facilitating the use of contraception does not lead to the immediate demise of the patient, unlike denial of a blood transfusion. Therefore, it makes sense to prevent a person from continuing to operate as a physician if he or she will refuse to provide necessary blood transfusions, but admitting this does not commit a person to holding that all doctors have a duty to facilitate abortion or contraception.

The argument that physicians should not be allowed to practice if they refuse to provide abortion procedures involves circular reasoning. Precisely at issue is whether performing abortions ought to be considered a central part of the role and responsibilities of the physician or health care provider. The question about what is or is not part of the role and responsibilities of a health care provider is simply another way of phrasing the question of whether there is a duty to perform abortions. Those who seek to protect conscience rights claim that willingness to perform an abortion is not a central part of the medical art and that it indeed contradicts the role and responsibilities of the physician. Those who wish to override conscientious claims of physicians deny this. Brock's appeal to it being a duty of physicians to care for patients merely begs the question.

According to Brock's view, a physician is required to provide certain services to patients: "This level of services should include all legal and beneficial medical interventions sought by patients."[17] But the debate in the medical community is precisely about whether abortion is a beneficial medical invention for patients. Refusing to perform an abortion is fully consistent with the goals of medicine, namely to restore or preserve health, for pregnancy is not a disease. In contrast, refusing to perform transfusions undermines the goal to restore health. Those in favor of abortion consider it a beneficial medical intervention; those opposed to abortion do not consider it to be beneficial because they believe that in such a case, a physician treats two patients, at least one of whom is lethally harmed by the procedure. The question is partly what counts as a benefit, but more importantly the issue is whose benefit counts, the mother's alone or also that of the developing human being within her.

Robert D. Orr's critique of his medical colleagues in the American College of Obstetricians and Gynecologists (ACOG) illustrates the division in the medical community between those for and those against conscience protection:

> ACOG erroneously maintains that negative patient autonomy (the right to refuse a recommended treatment) and positive patient autonomy (the right to demand a treatment) are morally equivalent. It is a well-established and longstanding tenet of medicine that the patient's right to refuse is nearly inviolable, but a patient's right to demand a specific treatment is subject to physician discretion and veto. Were this not so, patients could demand unnecessary surgery, and they would not require prescriptions for antibiotics or narcotics. Society has supported such professional refusals of procedures or drugs the physician believes to be deleterious to the patient based on patient beneficence. Similarly, society has until recently supported physician refusal based on his or her right of conscience."[18]

To hold that negative patient autonomy—the ability to refuse a recommended treatment—is absolute is not to say that positive patient autonomy—the right to demand a treatment—is absolute. Clearly, positive patient autonomy is not absolute. The right to refuse treatment, at least for mentally competent patients, admits scarcely any exceptions. The right to obtain requested treatments or services admits multiple exceptions such as "unnecessary surgery, and . . . prescriptions for antibiotics or narcotics."[19] If a doctor has the obligation simply to do whatever it is that a patient requests, regardless of the physician's medical judgment, then we have a radically different concept of the role of the physician than virtually any other society accepts. Scarcely anyone wants to force physicians to mutilate female genitalia, remove healthy limbs, assist in suicides, or participate in capital punishment, yet absolute positive patient autonomy would require such participation against the will of the physician.

Finally, critics of conscience protections, such as members of the ACOG, argue that health-care professionals should be obligated to tell patients about abortion and contraception, so as to ensure informed consent. The ACOG is not entirely consistent, however, about the importance of sharing information with patients. As Orr mentions, "Edmund

Pellegrino, chair of the President's Council on Bioethics, has noted the irony of this provision since the ACOG has gone to court to fight laws requiring abortion doctors to offer informed consent information to patients on the risks and alternatives to abortion."[20] In agreement with the ACOG, Thomas May and Mark P. Aulisio argue, "If we take informed consent seriously, we must limit conscience-based refusal to provide such information, since allowing refusal could deprive patients of even knowing what options exist."[21] It is logically possible that not mentioning the existence of contraception and abortion could—in some imaginary world—deprive patients of even knowing these options exist. Mentally handicapped adults may be unaware that abortion and contraception are options, but such persons cannot give informed consent. Children may be unaware that abortion and contraception are options, but they too cannot give informed consent (unless we suppose that they cannot give informed consent for sexual intercourse but can give informed consent to using contraceptives in sexual intercourse). In the United States, the percentage of adults capable of giving informed consent who are unaware that contraception and abortion are options is approaching zero. Among those possible few who are unaware of contraception and abortion are most likely people like the Amish who would not give informed consent to such practices anyway. Indeed, there are probably few treatments offered by doctors that are more well-known than contraception and abortion, so it is not very plausible to argue that there is a pressing need among patients to be informed of the possibility of using contraception or abortion. Given that both contraception and abortion are elective procedures, consistency would demand that patients also be informed of other elective procedures so as not to be deprived of informed consent. But no one holds that all doctors must inform all their patients of the possibilities of breast augmentation, botox injections, rhinoplasty, and facelifts. There is even less reason to inform patients about abortion or contraception because they are better known and, unlike most elective medical procedures, injurious to health understood in an objective sense.

Does informing a patient of legal options that other doctors would offer violate the obligation to help a patient develop a well-formed conscience? This question is an interesting one. First, it is not practical to hold that there is an obligation to inform a patient about *all* legal options. Providing an exhaustive list of all possible legal medical procedures would unreasonably burden both physician and patient. Should a doctor be obliged to inform patients about some medical procedures, such as abortion and contraception, but not others? It is difficult to see why abortion and contraception should be singled out for this preferential treatment, particularly in light of the fact that virtually all adults capable of giving informed consent to a medical procedure are highly likely aware that both abortion and contraception are legal options.

Informing someone of legal options such as abortion and contraception is not, however, necessarily cooperation with evil in a formal sense. It is difficult to imagine, but a lecture by a pro-life professor might inform an ignorant student that both contraception and abortion are legal, yet it would hardly be formal cooperation in wrongdoing should the student make use of that knowledge to get an abortion or use contraception. As material cooperation, informing someone of their legal options can be justified for a proportionately serious reason. Such disclosure about a procedure does not violate a well-formed conscience as would referral to such a specialist.

This chapter discusses a number of different approaches to the issue of conscience protection, but the following chapter treats the specific approach advocated by Bernard Dickens. Dickens provides a number of arguments articulated in a series of articles that challenge the idea that health care professionals have a right to act according to their consciences. The next chapter presents Dickens's challenges and attempts to answer them.

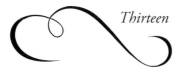

Thirteen

Conscientious Objection and Health Care

In several articles,[1] Bernard Dickens argues in favor of reducing or eliminating legal protection(s) for conscientiously objecting health-care workers and institutions. This chapter examines his arguments that (1) appeals to discrimination as a basis for conscientious objection are illegitimate, (2) conscientious objection undermines patients' rights and their autonomy, (3) doctors who conscientiously object to performing abortions have a duty to refer patients to physicians who are willing to provide abortions, (4) Kant's principle of respect for humanity as an end in itself is violated by conscientious objection to abortion, (5) remarks by Pope John Paul II support the contention that physicians should not conscientiously object to abortion, and (6) institutions, such as Catholic hospitals, have responsibilities that require them to provide abortions. Upon examination, none of these arguments establishes that health-care workers are not entitled to the prerogative of conscientiously objecting to performing or cooperating in the performance of abortion.

Appeals to Discrimination as a Basis for Conscientious Objection
are Illegitimate

Dickens's first argument against conscientious objection arises from an
assertion that anti-discrimination laws should not to be used as a basis for
conscientious objection to abortion:

> Protection against discrimination is in principle a legitimate goal
> of legislation, since discrimination is an act of superiority directed
> against those seen to be in an inferior position. Anti-discrimination
> laws are intended to relieve less powerful people from oppression by
> the more powerful. In this legislation, however, the protection is de-
> signed to privilege adherents primarily of a religious faith, and to
> exploit the dependency and inferior status of patients, primarily
> women, who want access to reproductive services. Enactment of laws
> to empower individuals to subordinate others to their preferences
> by denial of medically indicated care, especially when they enjoy a
> legal monopoly to provide, is an abuse of the anti-discrimination
> principle.[2]

Laws protecting conscientious objection to abortion, according to
Dickens's view, do not defend the weak (by his example, the women seeking abortion) but rather the strong (physicians and health-care personnel). The laws thereby reinforce rather than undermine oppression, particularly of vulnerable women seeking reproductive services.

There is a legal and an ethical aspect to Dickens's argument. Legally,
at least in the United States, reverse discrimination violates the law. In
Parents Involved in Community Schools v. Seattle School District No. 1, U.S.
Supreme Court Chief Justice Roberts wrote for the majority: "The way
to stop discrimination on the basis of race is to stop discriminating on the
basis of race" (551 U.S. 701 2007). *Regents of the University of California
v. Bakke* likewise endorsed the illegality of reverse discrimination.

Ethically, Dickens's understanding of discrimination is deeply controversial because it excludes, in principle, reverse discrimination. But it
seems plausible, at least in some cases, that reverse discrimination is pos-

sible. For example, a man who is fired from his job as a nurse solely because of his gender has been discriminated against, even if men are
considered generally more advantaged than women in his society. A white
person fired from her job at an organization exclusively serving African-
Americans simply because of her race has been treated unfairly, even if
whites are considered generally more advantaged than people of color in
her society. Unless we embrace the fallacy of division which attributes to
each part whatever is characteristic of the whole, we need not assume that
in every circumstance, every man (or white person) is advantaged and
every woman (or person of color) is disadvantaged. If we reject the fallacy
of division, then we ought not to exclude in principle the possibility of
reverse discrimination. We have grounds then for rejecting Dickens's understanding of discrimination.

Conscience protections do not primarily privilege adherents of a religious faith because they do not single out a particular religious faith, nor
do they fail to protect those who have no religious faith but object to a
practice based on nonreligious reasons. Neither do conscience protections
empower individuals to subordinate others to their preferences because
denial of abortion by a particular physician does not necessarily mean
that the doctor's preference (that the patient does not have an abortion at
all) will be realized. Finally, the conscientious physician as an individual
does not enjoy a legal monopoly to provide medical services. Rather, the
medical profession as a whole has this monopoly. So, the point about
medical monopoly would apply only if the entire medical profession re-
fused to perform abortions—which is not the case.

Conscientious Objection Undermines Patients' Rights and
Their Autonomy

In his second argument, Dickens opposes conscientious objection as incompatible with the rights of patients and as an imposition on their
autonomy. "In short, such legislation that protects religious, moral, or
ethical preferences deprives patients of many of their reproductive and
other rights, and often empowers health service providers and institutions
in effect to impose their will at patient's cost, including the cost of health

care."[3] According to this view, conscientious objection violates the rights of patients and imposes on patients a set of moral beliefs that they may not share.

Is Dickens correct that legal protection of conscientious objection is a sword used to force adherence to religious beliefs on those who do not share them? Put less dramatically, does conscientious objection to abortion in effect force women to continue their pregnancies until birth? The evidence is abundant that the actual, real world consequences of legal protection for conscientious objection do not lead to the unavailability of abortion. Pro-life physicians have not and cannot "in effect" impose their will on patients,[4] forcing them not to get abortions, as is evident from the 1.2 million abortions that occur each year in the United States and the fact that abortion is one of the most common American medical procedures, despite current legal protections for conscientious objection in the U.S. law.

But even if women can still get abortions from other providers, as the high incidence of abortion makes evident, surely conscientious objection by physicians imposes some cost upon women seeking abortion in terms of time and energy. If a doctor refuses to perform an abortion, then the patient who desires an abortion will have to find another doctor to perform the abortion.

However, similarly, if a particular doctor refuses to work on Saturday, then a patient who wants medical services from that doctor on Saturday will have to find another doctor. Likewise, if a doctor refuses to work without pay, then a patient who wants free medical care will have to seek out a doctor who will provide free medical care. Is it fair to say that such doctors who refuse to work on a particular day or refuse to provide free services "in effect impose their will at patient's cost, including the cost of health care"?[5] Such "imposition" is sometimes justified, for the interests of the patient should not always trump the interests of the physician. The interest of the doctor to act in an ethically conscientious way would seem to be a more important interest than a mere financial interest or an interest in not working on a particular day, so a fortiori the interests in protecting a physician's moral integrity is more than commensurate with the costs incurred by those seeking the denied service.

Suppose, however, that in a given situation, a doctor's refusal to perform an abortion did in fact lead to a particular woman not getting an abortion at all. Has this woman been denied what the law declares she is entitled to receive? Does conscientious objection, in this case, violate her rights?

If we are talking about legal rights, then it is false that conscientious objection violates patients' rights, at least in the United States, because patients do not have legal rights to force conscientiously objecting doctors to give them abortions. The Church Amendment, passed in 1973 shortly after the *Roe vs. Wade* decision, protects physicians from being forced to provide abortions. Does conscientious objection violate a patient's moral rights to abortion? To justify this conclusion, Dickens would need to provide an argument that abortion is morally permissible, but he offers no justification for this controversial assumption in the articles in question. If abortion is ethically impermissible—a case for this view is articulated in *The Ethics of Abortion: Women's Rights, Human Life, and the Question of Justice*[6]—then an appeal to the moral right to obtain an abortion is mistaken, for we cannot have a moral right to do what we have a moral duty not to do.

Suppose, for the sake of argument, that abortion is ethically permissible. Would physicians then have an ethical obligation to provide abortions in order not to violate the rights of women? An answer to this question depends upon whether one understands the moral right to abortion as a liberty right or as a claim right. Liberty rights, as defined earlier, involve the lack of a duty not to perform the act in question. An example of a liberty right includes the right to free speech. I may speak freely because I have no duty not to speak. A liberty right does not imply that others have duties to help me exercise my right. My right to free speech is not violated if the *New York Times* refuses to give me a biweekly op-ed column or if NBC does not broadcast my speeches. If abortion is a liberty right, then no doctor has a duty to perform an abortion because liberty rights create no duties for others to cooperate in what we are freely doing.

A claim right, in contrast, involves the duties of others to either refrain from some action or to aid us in some action. Our claim right not to be enslaved entails the duty of others not to enslave us. Our claim right to live is extensionally equivalent to the duty of others not to intentionally kill us. Our claim right to property necessitates the duty of others not to steal or destroy what belongs to us. So, one could argue, a woman's claim right to abortion entails the duty of her doctor to provide one. This view undermines conscientious objection.

This argument begs the question. Precisely at issue is whether doctors have an obligation to provide abortions. Therefore, to appeal to the premise that a woman has a claim right to receive an abortion from her doctor is simply another way of stating the conclusion that her doctor has a duty to perform abortion. The premise that is supposed to justify the conclusion simply restates the desired conclusion. The conclusion that doctors have a duty to provide abortions cannot be sustained by the premise that women have a claim right to abortion without engaging in circular reasoning.

Should not the physical needs of patients take precedence over the spiritual needs or ethical preferences of doctors? Dickens notes that health-care providers have a rich history of risking their own well-being for the good of their patients.[7] For example, they expose themselves to dangerous diseases in the course of treating patients. So too, Dickens reasons, they ought to sacrifice their own spiritual desires in order to perform certain tasks for the good of patients.

This argument fails to justify its conclusion in part because there is an important distinction between risking harm to oneself and certainly harming oneself. Doctors do have a strong tradition of risking their own well-being, but no one would suggest that doctors must certainly harm themselves for their patients' well-being (for example, by providing their nonduplicate organs to needy patients, by always providing patients free medical care, or by refusing to take vacations). A risk differs from a certainty. A conscientious objector performing an abortion certainly harms herself, minimally by harming her moral integrity. She does not merely risk harming herself as she would by treating infectious patients. Further, a long history of ethical reflection and witness—Socrates in the *Crito,* Aquinas in the *Summa Theologiae,* Kant in the *Groundwork of the Metaphysics of Morals,* and contemporary figures such as Dietrich Bonhoffer, Martin Luther King, Jr., and Nelson Mandela—testifies that spiritual or moral harm is more serious than physical harm. If physicians have no moral obligation to intentionally inflict physical sacrifices upon themselves in order to serve their patients, then how much less do physicians have an obligation to intentionally inflict moral sacrifices on themselves.

Conscientiously Objecting Doctors Have a Duty to Refer Patients for Abortion

Dickens holds that physicians who conscientiously object to abortions have a duty to refer patients for abortions elsewhere.

> The duty to refer in good faith is widely recognized as a condition of accommodating conscientious objection. Those who require respect for their own conscience cannot show disrespect for the different conclusions of others, including patients requesting medically indicated care in which the objectors decline to participate and of professional colleagues who do not object to provide such care.[8]

There are two arguments here. The first is an appeal to the authority of the masses, a weak argument that a duty to provide references to the patient is "widely recognized." Moreover, Dickens provides no evidence that this is true. Within living memory, prior to *Roe v. Wade,* it was widely recognized that abortion ought to be illegal and is incompatible with sound medical practice. The second argument appeals to the premise that respect for the consciences of others requires that one facilitate the conscientious choices of others. Dickens writes, "Those who invoke their own conscience to refuse participation in reproductive health services show equal respect for patients' consciences by referring them, in good faith, to sources of such services that do not conscientiously object to provide them."[9] Clearly, however, respect for the conscientious judgment of others does not require acting to facilitate the execution of these judgments. If this premise were true, then pro-choice advocates, such as Dickens, should facilitate pro-life physicians' conscientious refusal to refer for abortions. Similarly, pro-choice advocates should facilitate the criminalization of abortion, a goal conscientiously sought by pro-life advocates. To have respect for another's conscience means that one should refrain from manipulating, coercing, or otherwise attempting to force someone to change their beliefs, but it does not mean that one must cooperate, facilitate, or aid others in carrying out whatever actions they choose.

Elsewhere, Dickens offers other arguments that conscientiously objecting doctors have a legal and ethical duty to refer for abortions.[10] He notes that making a referral in and of itself does not mean that the physician who did so has aided in the abortion that the referred doctor will perform. The point seems to be that because the deed viewed as immoral only takes place after the referral and after discussions between the patient and her new doctor, the physician who provided the referral is absolved of responsibility for the procedure. Secondly, Dickens notes that the doctor providing the referral does not receive any payment from the doctor receiving the referral, so the referring doctor is not complicit in what the doctor performing the abortion does. Thus, concludes Dickens, there is an ethical or legal duty for physicians to refer patients to physicians who can honor their requests.

Receiving financial rewards from another may or may not confirm cooperation in his wrongdoing. Just because I am not paid for facilitating some person to do some action, it hardly follows that I am not ethically responsible for facilitating that action. If teenagers come to me and ask where they can buy alcohol so they can get drunk and race their cars, and I refer them to the corner grocery where the clerk never checks identification, then I have facilitated their wrongdoing. Thus, I (partially but not fully) share in the responsibility for their evil actions whether or not the teenagers tip me for providing the information and whether or not I converse with the clerk providing the alcohol. Whether or not the referring doctor is paid and whether or not the referring physician speaks to the doctor performing the abortion, the referring doctor is ethically responsible for cooperating with the actions performed.[11] Because his argument rests on false premises, Dickens offers no sound justification for the conclusion that health care professionals have a duty to refer others to obtain abortions.

Kant's Principle of Respect for Humanity as an End in Itself Is Violated by Conscientious Objection to Abortion

In justifying his view of the proper role of conscience, Dickens appeals to the Kantian principle that we are to "act in such a way that you treat humanity, whether in your own person or in the person of another, always at the same time as an end and never simply as a means."[12] Dickens argues that if consciously objecting health providers treat patients for whom they offer care as "objects or means to serve their own spiritual ends," then they are violating this Kantian principle. In Dickens's words, "If providers intend only to give treatment to patients, but not to care for or about patients, and sacrifice their patients' needs to their own spiritual comfort in invoking conscientious objection to deny or obstruct indicated healthcare, their instrumental use of patients is unethical."[13] This Kantian argument against conscientious objection contains questionable premises. There is no evidence whatsoever that Kant thought that abortion was ethically permissible, let alone that Kant would view refraining from abortion as ethically impermissible. Kant's views, according to detailed historical research,[14] support the conclusion that it is abortion itself, not refraining from abortion, that violates the principle: "Act so that you treat humanity, whether in your own person or in that of another, always as an end and never as a means only."[15]

Assuming for the sake of argument that abortion is morally permissible, would it violate the principle of respecting humanity as an end to refrain from helping another person obtain an abortion so as to not violate one's conscience? The answer to this question may be illuminated by considering a different question. Would it violate the principle of respecting humanity as an end if one refrained from performing an abortion unless one were paid for providing the abortion? Presumably, many doctors would not perform medical services unless they were paid, so do doctors use their patients as a means in charging for their services? Ceteris paribus, the answer is negative, for both parties freely agree to engage in an exchange—so neither party is using the other as if a human person were a mere thing. Rather, both parties are respecting the other's autonomy in coming to an agreement in exchange. Kant's principle is not about using people for financial ends (or spiritual ends) but rather about using people simply as a means.

What is it to use people simply as a means? One uses other people simply as a means when one treats them or makes use of them as if they were things or tools without respect for their dignity and autonomy. Examples of the principle include intentionally killing the innocent, in which a human person is destroyed as if he or she were a thing, and theft, in which another person's labor is treated as if the person were a slave or a tool. By contrast, not entering into a voluntary agreement with another is not a case of a violation of the principle of respect. This clarification of the Kantian principle makes it clear why the principle of respect is not violated in the case of refraining from performing or participating in abortion. The patient, making use of her autonomy, requests an abortion. The doctor, making use of his or her autonomy, declines the request. Neither has used the other simply as a means. The patient retains her autonomy to continue to seek an abortion or to change her mind. The doctor retains his or her autonomy to act in accordance with her best ethical and medical judgments. Just as a doctor can choose to not perform an abortion if he or she is not going to be paid, without "using" the patient just for money, so too a doctor can choose to not perform an abortion if doing so would violate his or her conscience, without "using" the patient for spiritual purposes.

Remarks by Pope John Paul II Support the Idea that Physicians Should Not Conscientiously Object to Abortion

Dickens enlists Pope John Paul II to craft an argument that there is a contradiction between papal teaching about respecting individual consciences and the Catholic practice of opposing abortion. Dickens views papal statements as a contradiction of the Vatican's opposition to definitions of "reproductive freedom" found in the United Nations International Conference on Women in Beijing in 1995. Dickens writes, "Conscientious objectors risk failing to heed his [Pope John Paul II's] warning, that "[i]ntolerance can also result from the recurring temptation to fundamentalism, which easily leads to serious abuses."[16]

The pope's views, properly understood, do not justify Dickens's conclusion. For example, the pope's statement about intolerance is not quoted in full, leaving the impression that the context had something to do with conscientious objection to abortion. In fact, the full quotation from John Paul II reads: "Intolerance can also result from the recurring temptation to fundamentalism, which easily leads to serious abuses such as the radical suppression of all public manifestations of diversity, or even the outright denial of freedom of expression. Fundamentalism can also lead to the exclusion of others from civil society; where religion is concerned, it can lead to forced 'conversions.'"[17] The context has nothing to do with the practice of medicine, let alone an implicit rejection of conscientious objection to abortion. Rather, the pope was speaking about forced religious conversion or suppression of freedom of expression. According to John Paul II's view, each individual's conscience should be respected by everyone else, and people must not attempt to impose their own views on others by means of manipulation, coercion, or force. Freedom of conscience, however, is not the same as freedom of behavior. Behavior, which includes even acts endorsed by conscience, must be limited by the rights of others as well as considerations of the public good.[18] In John Paul II's perspective, the rights of others include the right to life of human beings in utero. The quotation simply is not relevant to the position that Dickens advocates.

In three similar scholarly contributions,[19] Dickens makes appeal to a 1991 quotation from Pope John Paul II to justify annulling claims of conscientious objection to performing abortions. The papal quotation reads, "Freedom of conscience does not confer a right to indiscriminate recourse to conscientious objection. When an asserted freedom turns into license or becomes an excuse for limiting the rights of others, the State is obliged to protect, also by legal means, the inalienable rights of its citizens against such abuses."[20] Dickens interprets this statement as being in conflict with conscientious objection to abortion. The exact logic of the connection is never made clear—indeed, in all three articles it is simply insinuated—but the idea seems to be that if conscientious objection limits the ability of women to get abortions, then such objection abuses their legal rights to abortion.

Dickens's repeated invocation of John Paul II's quotation to oppose conscientious objection to abortion is a contextually irresponsible use of the text and a radical misunderstanding of the late pontiff's work. Only by misinterpreting each key term in the quotation—for instance, "freedom," "rights," and "state obligation"—in ways diametrically opposed to the understanding of these terms in the thought of John Paul II does the quotation provide a semblance of support for the view Dickens defends. It would be difficult to find anyone more opposed to abortion than the late pope,[21] and to enlist him in an effort to overturn conscientious objection is utterly unwarranted. According to John Paul II's view, it is not the conscientious objection to perform an abortion that violates the rights of others. It is rather the performance of abortions that violates the rights of others, namely the right to life of the unborn human beings whose lives are ended. Characteristic of John Paul's view of the relationship of morality, law, abortion, and conscience is the following passage from *Evangelium Vitae:*

> Certainly the purpose of civil law is different and more limited in scope than that of the moral law. But "in no sphere of life can the civil law take the place of conscience or dictate norms concerning things which are outside its competence," which is that of ensuring the common good of people through the recognition and defence of their fundamental rights, and the promotion of peace and of public morality. The real purpose of civil law is to guarantee an ordered social coexistence in true justice, so that all may "lead a quiet and peaceable life, godly and respectful in every way" (1 Tim. 2:2). Precisely for this reason, civil law must ensure that all members of society enjoy respect for certain fundamental rights which innately belong to the person, rights which every positive law must recognize and guarantee. First and fundamental among these is the inviolable right to life of every innocent human being. While public authority can sometimes choose not to put a stop to something which—were it prohibited—would cause more serious harm, it can never presume to legitimize as a right of individuals—even if they are the majority of

the members of society—an offence against other persons caused by the disregard of so fundamental a right as the right to life. The legal toleration of abortion or of euthanasia can in no way claim to be based on respect for the conscience of others, precisely because society has the right and the duty to protect itself against the abuses which can occur in the name of conscience and under the pretext of freedom.[22]

According to the pope's view, there is no moral right to abortion, so denying someone an abortion does not violate the person's moral rights. The pope's opposition to the legalization of abortion is also well-known, namely, that he advocates that there ought to be no legal right to abortion. Similarly, abortion cannot be understood, in his view, as a legitimate act of freedom: "To claim the right to abortion, infanticide and euthanasia, and to recognize that right in law, means to attribute to human freedom a perverse and evil significance: that of an absolute power over others and against others. This is the death of true freedom."[23] According to John Paul II's view, it is abortion—not failing to perform an abortion—that is a violation of the inalienable rights of others, and it is abortion, not failing to refer others for abortion, that ought to be a crime. Only by completely distorting the meaning of central terms as understood by the pope and by ignoring other aspects of John Paul II's thought can Dickens enlist the pontiff as an ally in his contention that conscientious refusal of abortion should not be protected.

Institutions, Such as Catholic Hospitals, Do Not Have Rights of Conscientious Objection

According to Dickens's view, hospitals have responsibilities entailing that they should be forced to provide abortions in some circumstances. "However, as a corporation, an artificial legal person, a hospital is not recognized to adhere to a religious faith. In terms of the Roman Catholic tradition, a hospital has no soul to be protected against the mortal sin of abortion. Accordingly, a health care facility such as a hospital cannot invoke conscientious objection to refuse to provide lawful services when a community has been induced to rely upon it for such services."[24] Because a hospital does not have a soul, Dickens argues, its soul cannot be undermined by abortion, so the hospital has a duty to perform abortions.

According to Catholic teaching, corporate persons such as hospitals indeed do not have souls, but this red herring is irrelevant to the issue at hand: the legal and ethical duties of institutions. Legally, the Church Amendment protects the rights of institutions in the United States, such as Catholic hospitals, from being forced to perform abortions, so there is no legal duty for institutions in this jurisdiction to perform abortions. Ethically, either corporate persons have ethical responsibilities or they do not. If they do not, then institutions such as hospitals have no duties to provide abortions or anything else, so Dickens's argument fails. If corporate persons do have ethical responsibilities, then we face the question—as we do with individual physicians—whether there is any sound, valid argument that corporate persons must perform abortions. As argued earlier, all the arguments made by Dickens in favor of forcing individual doctors to perform abortions are unsound; these arguments are no more sound when applied to corporate persons.

Corporate persons—institutions such as hospitals, businesses, schools, and governments—do have responsibilities and are therefore in a sense corporate moral agents. As such, they are bound by norms of justice. The leaders of such corporate moral agents have the responsibility to ensure that the duties and responsibilities of the institution are discharged. In managing an institution, individuals in positions of leadership, as well as those who are not, have obligations to follow the same basic rules of justice that govern individuals. They cannot in truth say, "I did not personally accomplish the injustices—but merely facilitated my underlings doing the injustices." If such a view were true, leaders who facilitated war crimes but did not personally "pull the trigger" would be excused from wrongdoing. But this is absurd. If abortion is the unjust killing of an innocent human person, then this injustice should not be done by an individual person or by a corporate person. If others do not agree with this view, they may found their own hospitals or abortion clinics. Even if abortion is morally permissible, it still may not be the case that corporate persons have duties to facilitate abortion, as was argued for individual persons. At issue, in part, is the freedom of association, which cannot be maintained if institutions dedicated to particular purposes—such as restoring health (objectively understood), fighting disease, and promoting life—are forcibly transformed into an institution working to contrary purposes.

In summary, none of Dickens's arguments establishes that health-care workers or institutions should not enjoy the prerogative of conscientiously objecting to abortion. First, appeals that conscientious objection is a type of discrimination are not reasonable because reverse discrimination is possible. Second, conscientious objection does not undermine the rights of patients or their autonomy. Third, conscientiously objecting doctors do not have a duty to refer patients for abortion. Fourth, Kant's principle of respect for humanity as an end in itself is not violated by conscientious objection to abortion; on the contrary, Kant's principle supports objection to abortion. Fifth, remarks by Pope John Paul II do not support the argument that physicians should not conscientiously object to abortion; to say otherwise is to abuse the meaning of the central terms used by the late pontiff. Finally, institutions, such as Catholic hospitals, do not have responsibilities to provide abortions, any more than do individual physicians.

Notes

Chapter 1.   Introduction

1. Pellegrino, Schulman, and Merrill, *Human Dignity and Bioethics;* Congregation for the Doctrine of the Faith, *Dignitas Personae.*

2. These negative evaluations of human dignity can have profound effects on the legal culture. For a helpful appraisal of an earlier and influential critique of human dignity, see Keown and Jones, "Surveying the Foundations of Medical Law."

3. Pinker, "The Stupidity of Dignity."

4. Ibid., 30.

5. Ibid.

6. Ibid.

7. Bingham, "Desmond Hatchett Fathers 21 Children by 11 Women before Turning 30."

8. For a further critique of Pinker's article, see Levin, "Indignity and Bioethics."

9. Ursin, "Personal Autonomy and Informed Consent."

10. Sulmasy, "Dignity and Bioethics," 473.

11. Ibid.

12. Waldron, "Dignity, Rank, and Rights," 30.

13. Pinker, "The Stupidity of Dignity," 28.

14. Marquis, "Review of Christopher Kaczor, *The Ethics of Abortion,*" 1.

15. Ibid.

16. Marquis, "Why Abortion is Immoral."

17. Kaczor, *The Ethics of Abortion,* 97.

18. Marquis, "Review of Christopher Kaczor, *The Ethics of Abortion,*" 1.

19. Liao, "The Basis of Human Moral Status," 168.

20. Varelius, "Minimally Conscious State," 42.

21. Liao, "The Basis of Human Moral Status," 167.

22. Varelius, "Minimally Conscious State," 47.

23. On this point, see also Knapp, "Species Inegalitarianism as a Matter of Principle."

24. Dixon, "Darwinism and Human Dignity."

Chapter 2.   Are All Species Equal in Dignity?

1. McMahan, "Eating Animals the Nice Way."

2. Cahoone, "Hunting as a Moral Good"; Bruckner, "Considerations on the Morality of Meat Consumption."

3. Jamieson, "The Rights of Animals and the Demands of Nature," 183.

4. Varelius, "Minimally Conscious State," 38.

5. An example of denial of equal human dignity is found in Bates, "Prenates, Postmorts, and Bell-Curve Dignity."

6. For arguments that birth is not a morally relevant characteristic, see Kaczor, *The Ethics of Abortion,* chapter 3.

7. Jamieson, "The Rights of Animals and the Demands of Nature," 183.

8. For some arguments that sentience, the capacity for desire, and self-consciousness are not necessary for basic moral status, see Kaczor, *The Ethics of Abortion,* chapters 4 and 2, sections 4.1.4, 4.1.1, and 2.4, respectively.

9. Singer, "Speciesism and Moral Status," 568.

10. Ibid., 571.

11. Neuhaus, *The Naked Public Square.*

12. Singer, "Speciesism and Moral Status," 574.

13. Kant, *Grounding for the Metaphysics of Morals,* 10.

14. Kain, "Kant's Defense of Human Moral Status," 66.

15. Ibid., 100.

16. See, for example, Cohen, "Contractarianism and Interspecies Welfare Conflicts."

17. Gunnarsson, "The Great Apes and the Severely Disabled," 312.

18. Kittay, "The Personal Is Philosophical Is Political," 623.

19. Singer, "Speciesism and Moral Status," 574.

20. See, for example, Reichmann, *Evolution, Animal "Rights," and the Environment.*

21. University of California–Santa Barbara neuroscientist Michael S. Gazzaniga emphasizes the vast, quantitative differences between humans taken collectively and all other species, including apes and chimps, taken collectively. The

differences in behavior are vast. Birthday parties, wedding showers, and luncheon receptions are utterly common for us, and utterly absent in every other species. Our physiology is also different. The human brain in not only proportionately bigger but also organized differently than these other species. It is not only a matter of brains but also other unique aspects of us humans that reflect a difference in rationality. See Gazzaniga, "Humans."

22. For some reflections on this subject, see Bruckner's remarks on animal overpopulation in his article "Considerations on the Morality of Meat Consumption."

23. Jamieson, "The Rights of Animals and the Demands of Nature," 185.

Chapter 3.   Equal Dignity and Equal Access to Fertility Treatments

1. Gelbaya, "Short- and Long-Term Risks to Women Who Conceive through In Vitro Fertilization."

2. See, for example, Porter, Peddie, and Bhattacharya, "Debate"; Smajdor, "Should IVF Guidelines Be Relaxed in the UK?"; Schmidt, "Should Men and Women Be Encouraged to Start Childbearing at a Younger Age?"

3. ASRM, "Access to Fertility Treatment by Gays, Lesbians, and Unmarried Persons," 1190.

4. Ibid. A similar defense is given about a related question in Murphy, "The Ethics of Helping Transgender Men and Women Have Children."

5. ASRM, "Access to Fertility Treatment by Gays, Lesbians, and Unmarried Persons."

6. Ibid., 1191.

7. Ibid.

8. Ibid.

9. Wilcox et al., "Why Marriage Matters," 11.

10. Popenoe and Whitehead, "Should We Live Together?" 2.

11. See, for example, Rhoads, *Taking Sex Differences Seriously;* Sax, *Why Gender Matters;* Moir and Jessel, *Brain Sex.*

12. See Prusak, "What Are Parents For?"

13. ASRM, "Access to Fertility Treatment by Gays, Lesbians, and Unmarried Persons," 1191.

14. Wardle, "The Potential Impact of Homosexual Parenting on Children."

15. Ibid., 841.

16. Stacey and Biblarz, "(How) Does the Sexual Orientation of Parents Matter?" 166.

17. Ibid., 171.

18. See Regnerus, "How Different Are the Adult Children of Parents Who Have Same-Sex Relationships?"

19. See, for example, Eckert et al., "Homosexuality in Monozygotic Twins Reared Apart."

20. Stacey and Biblarz, "(How) Does the Sexual Orientation of Parents Matter?" 170.

21. Ibid., 171.

22. Sprigg and Dailey, *Getting it Straight,* 103–8.

23. ASRM, "Access to Fertility Treatment by Gays, Lesbians, and Unmarried Persons," 1192.

24. John A. Robertson points out that according to existing ASRM guidelines, doctors are allowed to refuse fertility services if they think that the patient will not be adequate to the task of parenting. He also points out that existing ASRM guidelines were not followed in Nadya Suleman's case because she would have been eligible to have only one embryo implanted and not six. See Robertson, "The Octuplet Case." These guidelines conflict with the proposition that equal respect demands equal acquiescence to the requests of patients.

25. For more on this issue, see Porter, Peddie, and Bhattacharya, "Debate."

Chapter 4.   Procreative Beneficence

1. Savulescu and Kahane, "The Moral Obligation to Create Children with the Best Chance of the Best Life," 274.

2. I discuss cases of abortion for eugenic purposes elsewhere. See Smith and Kaczor, *Life Issues, Medical Choices,* 46–48.

3. Savulescu and Kahane, "The Moral Obligation to Create Children with the Best Chance of the Best Life," 278.

4. Strömberg et al., "Neurological Sequelae in Children Born after In-Vitro Fertilisation."

5. Hansen et al., "The Risk of Major Birth Defects After Intracytoplasmic Sperm Injection and In Vitro Fertilization," 725.

6. Hitti, "CDC: IVF May Boost Birth Defect Risk."

7. Savulescu and Kahane, "The Moral Obligation to Create Children with the Best Chance of the Best Life," 278, emphasis added.

8. Wilcox et al., "Why Marriage Matters," 12–31.

9. Savulescu and Kahane, "The Moral Obligation to Create Children with the Best Chance of the Best Life," 278.

10. Ibid., 281, emphasis added.

11. Davis, "The Parental Investment Factor and the Child's Right to an Open Future," 26.

12. As cited by Murphy, "Choosing Disabilities and Enhancements in Children," 44.

13. Singer, "Famine, Affluence, and Morality."

14. Bennett, "The Fallacy of the Principle of Procreative Beneficience," 271.

15. Ibid., 272.

16. Dekker, "The Illiberality of Perfectionist Enhancement."

17. Lewis, *The Abolition of Man,* 68–69.

18. Dekker, "The Illiberality of Perfectionist Enhancement," 94.

19. Savulescu and Kahane, "The Moral Obligation to Create Children with the Best Chance of the Best Life," 286.

20. Murphy, "Choosing Disabilities and Enhancements in Children," 48.

Chapter 5.   Embryo Adoption and Artificial Wombs

1. Oderberg, *Applied Ethics,* 5.

2. At Temple University, Dr. Aquinas Schaffer, Professor of Physiology and Pediatrics, has developed a synthetic amniotic fluid of oxygen-rich perflubron, an inert liquid that can carry more oxygen than blood can. (See Leach et al., "Partial Liquid Ventilation with Perflubron in Premature Infants with Severe Respiratory Distress Syndrome.") Most premature infants die because their lungs cannot receive sufficient oxygen, but Professor Schaffer's synthetic amniotic fluid could overcome this obstacle. He has tested the liquid on premature lamb fetuses who were successfully sustained using the artificial amniotic fluid after being transferred from their mothers' wombs. Lack of funding has thus far prevented tests on infants born prematurely. (See Zimmerman, "The Fetal Position.")

3. Dr. Hung Ching Liu, Professor of Reproductive Medicine in Clinical Obstetrics and Gynecology and Professor of Clinical Reproductive Medicine at Cornell University, has "taken steps toward developing an artificial womb by removing cells from the lining of a woman's womb and then, using hormones, growing layers of these cells on a model of a uterus. The model eventually dissolves, leaving a new artificial womb that continues to thrive. What's more, Liu's team found that within days of being placed in the new womb, embryos will attach themselves to its walls and being to grow. . . . [R]esearchers do not yet know how long after the beginning stages of gestation this artificial womb could be viable" (Zimmerman, "The Fetal Position," 15). If Dr. Liu's research is successful, these artificial wombs could be implanted in women whose uteruses have been

damaged or removed due to pathology, paving the way to reproductive success for many infertile women.

4. Dr. Yoshinori Kuwabara, Professor of Obstetrics and Gynecology at Juntendo University in Japan, has perhaps gone the furthest in developing external means of gestation. His team of researchers has constructed a clear acrylic tank about the size of a bread basket that is filled with a solution that functions as amniotic fluid and is stabilized at the appropriate body temperature. In this tank, they kept goat fetuses alive more than a week, attached through their umbilical cords to machines that function as placentas. Dr. Kuwabara has predicted that the use of artificial wombs for human beings could begin within the next five years. See Zimmerman, "Ectogenesis."

5. CDF, *Dignitas Personae*, 19.

6. CDF, *Donum Vitae*, I.6 and II.5, original emphasis removed.

7. John Paul II, *Evangelium Vitae*, 47.

8. CDF, *Donum Vitae*, II.B, 5.

9. Shettles, "Tubal Embryo Successfully Transplanted in Utero."

10. CDF, *Donum Vitae*, II.1.

11. Ibid., II.2.

12. Althaus, "Can One 'Rescue' a Human Embryo?" 115.

13. CDF, *Donum Vitae*, II.8.

14. Ibid., II.A, 1.

15. Tonti-Filippini, "The Embryo Rescue Debate," 124. For similar points, see Mary Geach's negative response to the question, in "Are There Any Circumstances in Which It Would Be Morally Admirable for a Woman to Seek to Have an Orphan Embryo Implanted in Her Womb?"

16. Aquinas, *Summa Theologiae*, III, q. 29, a. 2.

17. Stanmeyer, "An Embryo Adoptive Father's Perspective."

18. Brakman, "Stewards of Each Other."

19. Althaus, "Can One 'Rescue' a Human Embryo?"; Althaus, "Human Embryo Transfer and the Theology of the Body."

20. Pacholczyk, "Some Moral Contraindications to Embryo Adoption."

21. Brugger, "In Defense of Transferring Heterologous Embryos."

22. Ibid., 98.

23. Ibid.

24. Ibid.

25. CDF, *Donum Vitae*, II.3.

26. Ibid.

27. I leave to one side the interesting and important question of embryo adoption in which a woman who has had an embryo transferred to her uterus decides to place the child for adoption after birth. In other words, I am not address-

ing the permissibility of splitting gestational motherhood and social motherhood. Does a woman who adopts an embryo have an obligation also to rear the embryo as her child? If she cannot rear the child as her own, does she have an obligation to not become that child's gestational mother? For a thoughtful answer to these questions, see Brugger, "In Defense of Transferring Heterologous Embryos."

28. John Paul II, *Evangelium Vitae*, 63.

Chapter 6.   The Ethics of Ectopic Pregnancy

On February 7, 2007, a version of this paper was presented in Dallas, Texas, with the title "Ectopic Pregnancy and the Catholic Hospital," to a group of 170 bishops and ten cardinals from the United States, Canada, Mexico, Central America, the Caribbean, the Philippines, India, and Europe at the Twenty-First Workshop for Bishops. The workshop title was "Urged on by Christ: Catholic Health Care in Tension with Contemporary Culture."

1. Bowring, "The Moral Dilemma of Management Procedures for Ectopic Pregnancy," 101.

2. Pope John Paul II wrote: "[B]y the authority which Christ conferred upon Peter and his Successors, in communion with the Bishops—who on various occasions have condemned abortion and who in the aforementioned consultation, albeit dispersed throughout the world, have shown unanimous agreement concerning this doctrine—I declare that direct abortion, that is, abortion willed as an end or as a means, always constitutes a grave moral disorder, since it is the deliberate killing of an innocent human being" (*Evangelium Vitae*, 62).

3. Rock, *TeLinde's Operative Gynecology*, 420.

4. Some authors hold that salpingostomy is not intentional abortion. See, for example, Grisez, *Abortion: The Myths, the Realities, the Arguments*, 340–41; and Moraczewski, "Managing Tubal Pregnancies: Part 1," 1–4. Other authors believe that salpingostomy is intentional abortion. See, for example, Clark, "Methotrexate and Tubal Pregnancies: Direct or Indirect Abortion?"

5. For a discussion of this once debated case, see Connery, *Abortion*, 295–300.

6. Shettles, "Tubal Embryo Successfully Transplanted in Utero," 2026.

7. Wallace, "Transplantation of Ectopic Pregnancy from Fallopian Tube to Cavity of Uterus." It is possible that both cases can be explained through heterotopic pregnancy in which twins are carried simultaneously, one outside the uterus and one inside the uterus. This conjecture lacks evidence.

8. May writes: "I contend that it is morally imperative today to make every effort possible to discover and transplant into the uterus those unborn

babies who have, unfortunately, implanted in the fallopian tube or other ectopic sites and not in the uterus where they belong" ("The Management of Ectopic Pregnancies," 146). In his book *Catholic Bioethics and the Gift of Human Life*, May reverses his previous position on the use of methotrexate to treat ectopic pregnancy. He no longer views its use as intentionally killing the embryo.

9. In his article "Moral and Medical Considerations in the Management of Extrauterine Pregnancy," Diamond writes: "The long-term hoped-for solution to the dilemma will be the development of successful techniques for the transplantation of fetuses growing in ectopic location into the uterine cavity" (11).

10. Bowring writes: "This [transplantation technique] needs to be reconsidered and pursued, especially with the certainty that it is not just plausible, but possible. Convincing the medical field to focus on re-implantation is the true moral imperative in the issue of managing ectopic pregnancy today." "The Moral Dilemma of Management Procedures for Ectopic Pregnancy" (118).

11. May, "Methotrexate and Ectopic Pregnancy." For his more recent position, one that accepts the use of methotexate and salpingostomy, see May, *Catholic Bioethics and the Gift of Human Life*, 201–2.

12. I would like to thank T. Murphy Goodwin, MD, Chief of Maternal-Fetal Medicine at USC, as well as Bryron Calhoun, MD, the National Medical Advisor for the National Institute of Family and Life Advocates, who answered many of my questions about the medical practices discussed in this paper. An anonymous reviewer objected, noting, "The author has a problem . . . (of which he may not be aware) in characterizing salpingostomy as not being an attack on the embryo because it can be removed intact. The difficulty is that such a characterization relies on understanding the procedure as one done via laparotomy as opposed to laparoscopy. Laparoscopic salpingostomy does not allow the same sort of unimpeded access to the fallopian tube that laparotomy does. Since most procedures for unruptured ectopic pregnancy are now done laparoscopically, the procedure is often far less discriminating in how intact the embryo remains. [In a laparoscopic salpingostomy] the ectopic pregnancy is removed blindly without any concern for removing it as a discrete and intact entity. Perhaps this point could be addressed given the economic and medical pressures to perform this procedure laparoscopically." This consideration is important but it does implicitly presuppose what I was trying to show, that salpingostomy can be done (if performed via laparotomy) in such a way as to preserve the bodily integrity of the embryo. A laproscopic salpingostomy does not do this, but I address this case in the next paragraph of the body of this chapter.

13. Thomas Aquinas, *Summa Theologiae*, II-II, q. 64, a. 7.

14. See Ford, "The Morality of Obliteration Bombing."

15. United States Conference of Catholic Bishops, *Ethical and Religious Directives for Catholic Health Care Services,* directive 36, emphasis added.

16. Statistic cited by Cavagnaro, "Treating Ectopic Pregnancy: A Moral Analysis (Part II)," 4.

17. Morlock et al., "Cost-Effectiveness of Single-Dose Methotrexate Compared with Laparoscopic Treatment of Ectopic Pregnancy."

18. Physicians Vicken Sepilian and Ellen Wood write: "A bhCG level of greater than 15,000 IU/L, fetal cardiac activity, and free fluid in the cul-de-sac on US (presumably representing tubal rupture) are contraindications [for MXT]" ("Ectopic Pregnancy"). See also Barnhart et al., "The Medical Management of Ectopic Pregnancy."

19. Sepilian and Wood note: "embryonic cardiac motion can be observed 3.5–4 weeks postconception, about 5.5–6 weeks after the last menstrual period" ("Ectopic Pregnancy").

20. A number of ethicists have argued that the use of methotrexate is morally impermissible, for example, Charles E. Cavagnaro, Thomas W. Hilgers, and Bernard Nathanson. Others hold that its use to treat tubal pregnancy is permissible, for example, Albert Moraczewski, Benedict Ashley, Patrick Norris, and Peter Clark.

21. Although some experiments have been performed in which MXT is injected directly into the embryo, it should be noted that MXT is normally not administered directly upon the body of the embryo but rather is consumed orally by the woman or via injection into her body. Thus, even if "acting upon the body" of the embryo were morally dispositive for determining intentional effects as opposed to side effects, it is not relevant for the normal use of MXT.

22. Connery, *Abortion,* 162. As an anonymous reviewer helpfully noted, Raynaud himself thought the ectopic fetus was an unjust aggressor and that the distinction between "direct" and "indirect" was not relevant in such cases. Nevertheless, this colorfully illustrates the general principle that neither the certainty of the effect nor acting upon the body of another entails that a lethal effect which follows from the action must be intended.

23. Moraczewski, "Managing Tubal Pregnancies: Part 2," 4.

24. I argue this point further in my book *The Edge of Life,* chapter 6.

25. The rest of this paragraph is drawn virtually verbatim from one of the reader's reports.

26. Finnis, Grisez, and Boyle, "'Direct' and 'Indirect,'" 20.

27. May, "Methotrexate and Ectopic Pregnancy," 1–3.

28. These matters have been debated in other contexts. See Kaczor, "Intention, Foresight, and Mutilation."

29. Bowring, "The Moral Dilemma of Management Procedures for Ectopic Pregnancy," 109.

30. For example, Cavagnaro speaks of "the shared maternal-fetal organ of pregnancy—the placenta" ("Treating Ectopic Pregnancy: A Moral Analysis [Part II]," 4).

31. Connery, *Abortion,* 300.

32. Ibid., 177.

33. Finnis, Grisez, and Boyle, "'Direct' and 'Indirect,'" 28–29.

34. Kaczor, "Distinguishing Intention from Foresight."

35. For more, see Bratman, *Intention, Plans and Practical Reason;* Cavanaugh, *Double-Effect Reasoning,* 91–108.

36. I owe this insight to Alexander Pruss.

37. Shewmon, "The Dead Donor Rule: Lessons from Linguistics?" 293–95.

38. Tuohey, "The Implications of the *Ethical and Religious Directives for Catholic Health Care Services* on the Clinical Practice of Resolving the Ectopic Pregnancy," 46.

Chapter 7.   The Ethics of Fetal Surgery

1. Chervenak and McCullough, "Ethics of Fetal Surgery."

2. McCullough and Chervenak, *Ethics in Obstetrics and Gynecology,* 97–101.

3. Chervenak and McCullough, "Ethics of Fetal Surgery," 238.

4. Ibid.

5. For more on this topic, see Kaczor, *The Ethics of Abortion,* chapter 4, section 4.1.2.

6. Chervenak and McCullough, "Ethics of Fetal Surgery," 238.

7. Ibid., 241–42.

8. Ibid., 242.

9. Ville, "Fetal Therapy: Practical Ethical Considerations," 624.

10. Ibid., 623.

11. Ibid.

12. Garcia, "The Doubling Undone? Double Effect in Recent Medical Ethics," 245.

13. Ville, "Fetal Therapy: Practical Ethical Considerations," 624.

14. For a philosophical discussion of the gradualists/developmental view, see Kaczor, *The Ethics of Abortion.* On the developmental view and why it is mistaken, see chapter 4, section 4.3 of this book. See, too, my article "Equal Rights, Unequal Wrongs."

15. Ville, "Fetal Therapy: Practical Ethical Considerations," 624

16. Ruth Padawer, "The Two-Minus-One Pregnancy."

17. Saletan, "Half-Aborted."

18. Ibid.

19. For the medical background see, for example, Chmaita and Quintero, "Operative Fetoscopy in Complicated Monochorionic Twins"; and Rossi and D'Addario, "Umbilical Cord Occlusion for Selective Feticide in Complicated Monochorionic Twins."

20. See, for example, Finnis, Grisez, and Boyle, "'Direct' and 'Indirect.'"

Chapter 8.   The Violinist Argument Revisited

1. For a summary of numerous attempts to justify abortion and why these attempts fail, see Kaczor, *The Ethics of Abortion.*

2. Kissling, "Abortion Rights Are under Attack, and Pro-Choice Advocates are Caught in a Time Warp."

3. Manninen, "Rethinking *Roe v. Wade.*"

4. Ibid., 39.

5. Ibid.

6. Ibid., 40.

7. Marquis, "Manninen's Defense of Abortion Rights Is Unsuccessful," 56.

8. This is disputed by Elizabeth Brake, who argues that because mothers do not have obligations to their unborn children, neither do fathers have obligations to provide child support. See her article, "Fatherhood and Child Support: Do Men Have a Right to Choose?"

9. Rajczi, "Abortion, Competing Entitlements, and Parental Responsibility," 391.

10. Ibid., 388.

11. Manninen, "Rethinking *Roe v. Wade,*" 43.

12. As Rosalind Hursthouse points out, in the violinist case, "I cannot do my job, I cannot go visit my sick mother, I cannot go to my sister's wedding, I cannot go to films, I cannot go swimming, I cannot read (well, perhaps the violinist is a great talker), I cannot have a confidential conversation with anyone and I cannot make love. And all of this for a whole nine months. But the usual pregnancy does not make one bed-ridden, and even when it does, very rarely for nine months; nor is the fetus, even assuming it to be a person, someone whose presence rules out reading, private conversations, and sex" (*Beginning Lives,* 203).

13. For a discussion of the link between abortion with parental duties, see Prusak, "Breaking the Bond: Abortion and the Grounds of Parental Obligations."

14. Chopra, "Childless Couples Look to India for Surrogate Mothers."

15. Grall, "Support Providers 2002: Household Economic Studies," 2.

16. See Finnis, "The Rights and Wrongs of Abortion."

17. Hopkins, "Can Technology Fix the Abortion Problem?" 317.

18. Walters and Dale, "DA: West Philadelphia Abortion Doctor killed 7 Babies with Scissors."

19. Hopkins, "Can Technology Fix the Abortion Problem?" 318.

20. O'Brien, "Can We Talk about Abortion?"

Chapter 9.   Faith, Reason, and Physician-Assisted Suicide

1. Engelhardt, "Physician-Assisted Suicide,"147.

2. John Paul II, *Evangelium Vitae,* 65, emphasis in the original.

3. Second Vatican Council, *Lumen Gentium,* 25.

4. Thomasma, "Assisted Death and Martyrdom," 135.

5. Ibid., 136.

6. Ibid.

7. Anselm, *Basic Writings,* 208.

8. White, *Grounds of Liability,* 83; Aulisio, "On the Importance of the Intention/Foresight Distinction," 192.

9. Quinn, "Actions, Intentions, and Consequences"; Cavanaugh, "The Intended/Foreseen Distinction's Ethical Relevance," 118–63.

10. S. Brock, "The Use of *Usus* in Aquinas' Psychology of Action."

11. Aquinas, *Summa Theologiae,* I-II, q. 20. a. 4.

12. Fuchs, "Gott—Der Herr über Leben und Tod."

13. Aquinas, *Summa Theologiae,* I-II, q. 98, a. 6.

14. Thomasma, "Assisted Death and Martyrdom," 138.

15. Ibid., 129.

16. Ibid., 130.

17. Aquinas held that within distributive justice, a just ruler may allot punishments and penalties for wrongdoing without undermining the love due to the one being punished. In fact, punishment within this sphere of justice can be an act of love for the community as well as for the criminal, to whose freedom the community, acting through the just ruler, responds appropriately. For more on this topic see Kaczor, "Capital Punishment and the Catholic Tradition."

18. Elsewhere, in Rom. 2:14–16, we read: "Indeed, when Gentiles, who do not have the law, do by nature things required by the law, they are a law for themselves, even though they do not have the law, since they show that the requirements of the law are written on their hearts, their consciences also bearing witness, and their thoughts now accusing, now even defending them."

19. Augustine, *On Christian Doctrine*, 544–45, 554–56.

20. Engelhardt, "Physician-Assisted Suicide," 148.

21. Bonaventure, *Disputed Questions on the Knowledge of Christ*, Aquinas, *Summa Theologiae*, I, q. 85; Plantinga, *Warrant and Proper Function*.

22. Engelhardt, "Physician-Assisted Suicide," 143–44.

23. Hobbes, *The English Works*, 116; Locke, *The Second Treatise on Government*, paragraphs 6 and 23.

24. "Wenn er, um einem beschwerlichen Zustande zu entfliehen, sich selbst zerstört, so bedient er sich einer Person, bloß als eines Mittels, zu Erhaltung eines erträglichen Zustandes bis zu Ende des Lebens. Der Mensch aber ist keine Sache, mithin nicht etwas, das bloß als Mittel gebraucht werden kann, sondern muß bei allen seinen Handlungen jederzeit als Zweck an sich selbst betrachtet werden" (Kant, *Grundlegung zur Metaphysik der Sitten*, 61).

25. Mill, *Utilitarianism*, 22.

26. See Keown, *Euthanasia, Ethics and Public Policy*.

Chapter 10.   PVS Patients and Pope John Paul II

1. Second Vatican Council, *Lumen Gentium*, 25.

2. O'Rourke, "Reflections on the Papal Allocution Concerning Care for Persistent Vegetative State Patients."

3. For those who deny such changes, see, for example, Dulles, "Religious Freedom: Innovation and Development"; Mullady, "Religious Liberty: Homogeneous or Heterogeneous Development?"; and, on usury, Finnis, *Aquinas*, 205–17.

4. Bretzke, "A Burden of Means: Interpreting Recent Catholic Magisterial Teaching on End-of-Life Issues."

5. Pope John Paul II, *Veritatis Splendor*, 80 et passim.

6. Bretzke, "A Burden of Means: Interpreting Recent Catholic Magisterial Teaching on End-of-Life Issues," 194. This claim is also found in Harvey, "The Burdens-Benefits Ratio Consideration for Medical Administration of Nutrition and Hydration to Persons in the Persistent Vegetative State," 103.

7. Harvey, "The Burdens-Benefits Ratio Consideration for Medical Administration of Nutrition and Hydration to Persons in the Persistent Vegetative State," 104. Making a similar point is Clark, "Tube Feedings and Persistent Vegetative State Patients: Ordinary or Extraordinary Means?" 57.

8. Orr, "Ethics and Life's Ending."

9. May, "Caring for Persons in the 'Persistent Vegetative State' and Pope John Paul II's March 20, 2004, Address 'On Life-Sustaining Treatments and the Vegetative State.'"

10. Harvey, "The Burdens-Benefits Ratio Consideration for Medical Administration of Nutrition and Hydration to Persons in the Persistent Vegetative State," 105.

11. See Garcia, "A Catholic Perspective on the Ethics of Artificially Providing Food and Water."

12. See, for example, Drane, "Stopping Nutrition and Hydration Technologies"; Harvey, "The Burdens-Benefits Ratio Consideration for Medical Administration of Nutrition and Hydration to Persons in the Persistent Vegetative State"; O'Rourke, "Reflections on the Papal Allocution Concerning Care for Persistent Vegetative State Patients"; Shannon, "Nutrition and Hydration: An Analysis of the Recent Papal Statement in Light of the Roman Catholic Bioethical Tradition."

13. Cahill, "Catholicism, Death and Modern Medicine."

14. Aquinas, *Summa Theologiae,* II-II, q. 10, a. 12.

15. Noonan's *Contraception* is an influential record of the condemnation, spread over many centuries, places, and theological approaches.

16. I do not view Pope John Paul II's teaching as inconsistent with tradition although I think it is a development. See Kaczor, "Capital Punishment and the Catholic Tradition."

17. O'Rourke, "Reflections on the Papal Allocution Concerning Care for Persistent Vegetative State Patients," 91.

18. Cahill, "Catholicism, Death and Modern Medicine," 17.

19. Garcia, "A Catholic Perspective on the Ethics of Artificially Providing Food and Water."

20. Clark, "Tube Feedings and Persistent Vegetative State Patients: Ordinary or Extraordinary Means?" 62; Cahill, "Catholicism, Death and Modern Medicine," 17.

Chapter 11.   Organ Donation after Cardiac Death

1. Verheijde, Rady, and McGregor, "Recovery of Transplantable Organs after Cardiac or Circulatory Death," 1.

2. Harter, "Overcoming the Organ Shortage."

3. Gardiner and Riley, "Non-Heart-Beating Organ Donation," 431.

4. Bell, "Non-Heart Beating Organ Donation," 177.

5. Verheijde, Rady, and McGregor, "Recovery of Transplantable Organs after Cardiac or Circulatory Death," 1.

6. Shewmon, "Brain Death: Can It Be Resuscitated?"

7. Miller and Truog, "The Incoherence of Determining Death by Neurological Criteria."

8. Kootstra, Daemen, and Oomen, "Categories of Non-Heart-Beating Donors."

9. Zeiler et al., "The Ethics of Non-Heart-Beating Donation," 528. According to this approach, the individual's decision whether or not to be an organ donor takes precedence over the recipient's need, but in cases in which there is no consent either for or against donation, the presumption is that the person would consent to organ donation and donation is performed unless the family objects.

10. Valko, "Ethical Implications of Non-Heart-Beating Organ Donation," 109.

11. Steinberg, "The Antemortem Use of Heparin in Non-Heart-Beating Organ Transplantation," 22.

12. Childress, "Non-Heart-Beating Donors of Organs," 204.

13. Ibid., 210.

14. Ibid., 211.

15. Ibid., 215.

16. Keown, "The Legal Revolution: From 'Sanctity of Life' to 'Quality of Life' and 'Autonomy.'"

17. University of Pittsburgh, "University of Pittsburgh Medical Center Policy and Procedure Manual," A5.

18. Clark and Deshmukh, "Non-Heart-Beating Organ Donation and Catholic Ethics," 544.

19. Steinberg, "The Antemortem Use of Heparin in Non-Heart-Beating Organ Transplantation."

20. Ibid., 22.

21. Bell, "Non-Heart Beating Organ Donation," 179; Steinberg, "The Antemortem Use of Heparin in Non-Heart-Beating Organ Transplantation," 19.

22. Steinberg, "The Antemortem Use of Heparin in Non-Heart-Beating Organ Transplantation," 20.

23. Pascal, *Oeuvres Complètes,* 398–99.

24. Steinberg, "The Antemortem Use of Heparin in Non-Heart-Beating Organ Transplantation," 20.

25. Zeiler et al., "The Ethics of Non-Heart-Beating Donation," 527.

26. For an extremely interesting take on the question, one sensitive to linguistic and cultural context, see Shewmon, "The Dead Donor Rule: Lessons from Linguistics?"

27. Bernat, Culver, and Gert, "On the Definition and Criterion of Death"; Shewmon, "The Brain and Somatic Integration," 458.

28. Bernat, *Ethical Issues in Neurology,* 113–43.

29. For a critique, see Lee and George, *Body-Self Dualism in Contemporary Ethics and Politics.*

30. National Conference of Commissioners on Uniform State Laws, Uniform Determination of Death Act, 1980.

31. Some might question why God cannot do what is logically impossible (thereby making room for the possibility that reversal of function is logically impossible and that God could have done it anyway). Aquinas argues that God cannot do what is logically impossible, such as to make square circles, to create another God, or both to give and not to give human beings free will at the same time and in the same respect. It is not as if God must consult with some celestial logic textbook which bans the Almighty from performing these works. Rather, the being of a thing, if it exists, exists ultimately because it is willed by God. So, for some being to exist and also not exist at the same time and in the same respect would involve God's willing and not willing the very same thing at the very same time and in the very same respect. It is, of course, possible for human beings to have divided wills, but God, according to Aquinas's understanding, is a perfect unity. God's will is one, and God does not contradict Himself. Thus, God cannot do that which is logically impossible, that which violates the law of non-contradiction: a thing cannot be and not be at the same time and in the same respect.

32. DuBois, "Non-Heart-Beating Organ Donation," 127.

33. DuBois, "Avoiding Common Pitfalls in the Determination of Death," 554.

34. Aristotle, *Categories,* in *The Complete Works of Aristotle,* 1:22.

35. Verheijde, Rady, and McGregor, "Recovery of Transplantable Organs after Cardiac or Circulatory Death," 3.

36. Capron, "The Bifurcated Legal Standard for Determining Death: Does It Work?" 132.

37. DuBois, "Avoiding Common Pitfalls in the Determination of Death," 554.

38. Shewmon, "Brainstem Death, Brain Death, and Death," 45.

39. Ben-David et al., "Survival after Failed Intraoperative Resuscitation."

40. DuBois, "Avoiding Common Pitfalls in the Determination of Death," 554.

41. These remarks are slightly different from, though inspired by, Shewmon, "The Dead Donor Rule: Lessons from Linguistics?" 294–96.

42. Herdman, Beauchamp, and Potts, "The Institute of Medicine's Report on Non-Heart-Beating Organ Transplantation," 86.

43. Grasser, "Donation after Cardiac Death: Major Ethical Issues," 541.

44. Carlberg, "Transplanting Lungs from Non-Heart-Beating Donors," 378.

45. Stanford University School of Medicine, "Deceased Donor as a Source of Organs for Heart Transplantation."

Chapter 12.   Conscience Protection and the Incompatibility Thesis

1. Mattox and Bowman, "Your Conscience, Your Right," 188.

2. Wicclair, "Is Conscientious Objection Incompatible with a Physician's Professional Obligations?" 171.

3. Ibid., 172.

4. Wicclair, "Conscience-Based Exemptions for Medical Students," 39.

5. Gerrard, "Is It Ethical for a General Practitioner to Claim a Conscientious Objection When Asked to Refer for Abortion?" 601.

6. United States Conference of Catholic Bishops, "The Catholic Church in America—Meeting Real Needs in Your Neighborhood," 12.

7. Wicclair, "Is Conscientious Objection Incompatible with a Physician's Professional Obligations?" 173.

8. Ibid., 176.

9. Ibid., 181.

10. Ibid.

11. Ibid., 183.

12. Ibid.

13. D. Brock, "Conscientious Refusal by Physicians and Pharmacists."

14. Ibid., 190.

15. Ibid., 191.

16. Kaczor, *The Ethics of Abortion,* 185–91.

17. D. Brock, "Conscientious Refusal by Physicians and Pharmacists," 191.

18. Orr, "Medical Ethics and the Faith Factor: The Endangered Right of Conscience," 53.

19. Ibid.

20. Ibid., 54.

21. May and Aulisio, "Personal Morality and Professional Obligations," 32.

Chapter 13.   Conscientious Objection and Health Care

1. Dickens, "Conscientious Objection: A Shield or a Sword?"; Cook, Olaya, and Dickens, "Healthcare Responsibilities and Conscientious Objection";

Dickens, "Legal Protection and Limits of Conscientious Objection"; Dickens, "Conscientious Objection and Professionalism."

2. Dickens, "Legal Protection and Limits of Conscientious Objection," 340.

3. Ibid.

4. Dickens, "Conscientious Objection: A Shield or a Sword?" 338, 346.

5. Dickens, "Legal Protection and Limits of Conscientious Objection," 340.

6. Dickens repeatedly describes the pro-life position by means of offensive, question-begging epithets such as: "a fundamentalist opinion of the point at which unborn human life warrants protection." See "Legal Protection and Limits of Conscientious Objection," 341. Dickens provides no argument for his assertion that not all human life should be protected and appears to think that such a view must be grounded in religious belief, though this assertion is not justified through argumentation. A refutation of the view that opposition to abortion must rely on theological or religious justification is provided by my book *The Ethics of Abortion,* as well as in many other philosophical works defending the pro-life position, including Patrick Lee's *Abortion and Unborn Human Life* and Robert P. George and Christopher Tollefsen's *Embryo: A Defense of Human Life,* to name only a few.

7. Dickens, "Legal Protection and Limits of Conscientious Objection," 346.

8. Ibid.

9. Dickens, "Conscientious Objection: A Shield or a Sword?" 345.

10. Dickens, "Conscientious Objection and Professionalism," 97.

11. Dickens, "Legal Protection and Limits of Conscientious Objection," 346. Dickens does not exhibit a nuanced understanding of Catholic teaching on cooperation with evil. He fails to elucidate the elementary distinctions between "material" and "formal" cooperation, asserting incorrectly that "Catholic doctrine on complicity makes it as illicit to facilitate a wrong as to commit it . . . ." ("Conscientious Objection: A Shield or a Sword?" 344). This assertion is true only in terms of formal cooperation, not in terms of most material cooperation; see Smith and Kaczor, *Life Issues, Medical Choices,* 133–36.

12. Kant, *Grounding for the Metaphysics of Morals,* 36.

13. Dickens, "Legal Protection and Limits of Conscientious Objection," 346.

14. Kain, "Kant's Defense of Human Moral Status."

15. Dickens notes that Kant's works were on the Index of Forbidden Books prior to the Second Vatican Council, and he insinuates that this means that the Catholic Church disagreed with Kant's principle that we ought not to use humanity in ourselves or others merely as a means, but rather always to respect them as ends. This is unfair. This Kantian principle, even before the Second Vatican Council, was widely endorsed in Catholic circles as is evident, for example, in the ethical writings of Bishop Karol Wojtyla, who later became Pope

John Paul II. Kant's philosophy, from a Catholic perspective, is in many ways erroneous, but not on this point.

16. Dickens, "Legal Protection and Limits of Conscientious Objection," 347.

17. Pope John Paul II, "If You Want Peace, Respect the Conscience of Every Person," 4.

18. John Paul II, *Veritatis Splendor,* 44: "The force of law consists in its authority to impose duties, to confer rights and to sanction certain behavior."

19. Dickens, "Conscientious Objection: Shield or Sword?" 337; Dickens, "Legal Protection and Limits of Conscientious Objection," 343; and Cook, Olaya, and Dickens, "Healthcare Responsibilities and Conscientious Objection," 252.

20. Pope John Paul II, "If You Want Peace, Respect the Conscience of Every Person," 24.

21. In *Evangelium Vitae,* 62, the pope wrote, "by the authority which Christ conferred upon Peter and his Successors, in communion with the Bishops—who on various occasions have condemned abortion and who in the aforementioned consultation, albeit dispersed throughout the world, have shown unanimous agreement concerning this doctrine—I declare that direct abortion, that is, abortion willed as an end or as a means, always constitutes a grave moral disorder, since it is the deliberate killing of an innocent human being. This doctrine is based upon the natural law and upon the written Word of God, is transmitted by the Church's Tradition and taught by the ordinary and universal Magisterium. No circumstance, no purpose, no law whatsoever can ever make licit an act which is intrinsically illicit, since it is contrary to the Law of God which is written in every human heart, knowable by reason itself, and proclaimed by the Church."

22. John Paul II, *Evangelium Vitae,* 71.

23. Ibid., 20.

24. Dickens, "Conscientious Objection and Professionalism," 99; see too, Cook, Olaya, and Dickens, "Healthcare Responsibilities and Conscientious Objection," 250.

Bibliography

Althaus, Catherine. "Can One 'Rescue' a Human Embryo? The Moral Object of the Acting Woman." *National Catholic Bioethics Quarterly* 5.1 (2005): 113–41.

———. "Human Embryo Transfer and the Theology of the Body." In *The Ethics of Embryo Adoption and the Catholic Tradition,* edited by Sarah-Vaughan Brakman and Darlene Fozard Weaver, 43–67. Dordrecht: Springer, 2007.

Anderson, Robert. "Boyle and the Principle of Double Effect." *American Journal of Jurisprudence* 52 (2007): 259–72.

Anselm. *Basic Writings: Proslogium, Monologium, Cur Deus Homo, Gaunilo's in Behalf of the Fool.* New York: Open Court Classics, 1962.

Aquinas, Thomas. *On Evil: Quaestiones Disputatae De Malo.* Edited by Jean Oesterle. Notre Dame: University of Notre Dame Press, 1995.

———. *Summa Theologiae in Opera Omnia Iussa Edita Leonis XIII P.M.* Rome: Ex Typographia Plygotta S.C. de Propaganda Fide, 1888–1906.

Aristotle. *The Complete Works of Aristotle: The Revised Oxford Translation.* Vol. 1. Edited by Jonathan Barnes. Princeton: Princeton University Press, 1984.

ASRM (Ethics Committee of the American Society for Reproductive Medicine). "Access to Fertility Treatment by Gays, Lesbians, and Unmarried Persons." *Fertility and Sterility* 92.4 (2009): 1190–93.

Augustine. *On Christian Doctrine.* Nicene and Post-Nicene Fathers 2. Grand Rapids, MI: Eerdmans, 1988.

———. *On the Morals of the Catholic Church.* Nicene and Post-Nicene Fathers 4. Grand Rapids, MI: Eerdmans, 1989.

Aulisio, Mark P. "On the Importance of the Intention/Foresight Distinction." *American Catholic Philosophical Quarterly* 70.2 (1996): 189–205.

Barnhart, K. T., G. Gosman, R. Ashby, and M. Sammel. "The Medical Management of Ectopic Pregnancy: A Meta-Analysis Comparing 'Single Dose' and 'Multidose' Regimens." *Obstetrics and Gynecology* 101.4 (2003): 778–84.

Bates, Stephen. "Prenates, Postmorts, and Bell-Curve Dignity." *Hastings Center Report* 38.4 (2008): 21–25.

Bell, M. D. D. "Non-Heart Beating Organ Donation: Old Procurement Strategy—New Ethical Problems." *Journal of Medical Ethics* 29.3 (2003): 176–81.

Ben-David, Bruce, Vincent C. Stonebraker, Robin Hershman, Christopher L. Frost, and H. Kenneth Williams. "Survival after Failed Intraoperative Resuscitation: A Case of 'Lazarus Syndrome.'" *Anesthesia & Analgesia* 92.3 (2001): 690–92.

Benedict Guevin, OSB, and Martin Rhonheimer. "On the Use of Condoms to Prevent Acquired Immune Deficiency Syndrome." *National Catholic Bioethics Quarterly* 5.1 (2005): 40–48.

Bennett, Rebecca. "The Fallacy of the Principle of Procreative Beneficence." *Bioethics* 23.5 (2009): 265–73.

Bernat, James. *Ethical Issues in Neurology*. Boston: Butterworth-Heinemann, 1994.

Bernat, James, Charles M. Culver, and Bernard Gert. "On the Definition and Criterion of Death." *Annals of Internal Medicine* 94 (1981): 389–94.

Bingham, John. "Desmond Hatchett Fathers 21 Children by 11 Women before Turning 30." *Telegraph* (London). May 29, 2009. http://www.telegraph.co.uk/news/worldnews/northamerica/usa/5404674/Desmond-Hatchett-fathers-21-children-by-11-women-before-turning-30.html.

Bonaventure. *Disputed Questions on the Knowledge of Christ*. Translated by Zachary Hayes. New York: Francisco Institute St. Bonaventure University, 1992.

Bowring, Kelly. "The Moral Dilemma of Management Procedures for Ectopic Pregnancy." In *Life and Learning 12: Proceedings of the Twelfth University Faculty for Life Conference at Ave Maria Law School 2002,* edited by Joseph W. Koterski, SJ, 97–126. Washington, DC: University Faculty for Life, 2003.

Boyle, Joseph. "Contraception and Anesthesia: A Reply to James Dubois." *Christian Bioethics* 14.2 (2008): 217–25.

———. "Cooperation and Integrity: How to Think Clearly about Moral Problems of Cooperation." In *Issues for a Catholic Bioethic,* edited by Luke Gormally, 187–99. London: The Linacre Centre, 1999.

———. "Double Effect and a Certain Type of Embryotomy." *Irish Theological Quarterly* 44.4 (1977): 303–18.

———. "Just War Doctrine and the Military Response to Terrorism." *Journal of Political Philosophy* 11.2 (2003): 153–70.

———. "Medical Ethics and Double Effect: The Case of Terminal Sedation." *Theoretical Medicine and Bioethics* 25.1 (2004): 51–60.

Boyle, Joseph, and Thomas Sullivan. "The Diffusiveness of Intention Principle: A Counter-Example." *Philosophical Studies* 31 (1977): 357–60.

Brake, Elizabeth. "Fatherhood and Child Support: Do Men Have a Right to Choose?" *Journal of Applied Philosophy* 22.1 (2005): 55–73.

Brakman, Sarah-Vaughan. "Stewards of Each Other: Catholic Social Thought and the Ethics of Embryo Adoption." In *The Ethics of Embryo Adoption and the Catholic Tradition,* edited by Sarah-Vaughan Brakman and Darlene Fozard Weaver, 119–38. Dordrecht: Springer, 2007.

Bratman, Michael. *Intention, Plans, and Practical Reason.* Cambridge, MA: Harvard University Press, 1987.

Bretzke, James T., SJ. "A Burden of Means: Interpreting Recent Catholic Magisterial Teaching on End-of-Life Issues." *Journal of the Society of Christian Ethics* 26.4 (2006): 183–200.

Brock, Dan W. "Conscientious Refusal by Physicians and Pharmacists: Who Is Obligated to Do What, and Why?" *Theoretical Medicine and Bioethics* 29.3 (2008): 187–200.

Brock, Stephen L. "On (Not Merely) Physical Objects of Moral Acts." *Nova et Vetera English Edition* 6.1 (2008): 1–62.

———. "The Use of *Usus* in Aquinas' Psychology of Action." In *Moral and Political Philosophy in the Middle Ages: Proceedings of the Ninth International Congress of Medieval Philosophy,* edited by B. Bazán, E. Andújar, and L. Sbrocchi, 654–64. Ottawa: Legas, 1992.

Brown, Brandon, and Jason Eberl. "Ethical Considerations in Defense of Embryo Adoption." In *The Ethics of Embryo Adoption and the Catholic Tradition,* edited by Sarah-Vaughan Brakman and Darlene Fozard Weaver, 103–40. Dordrecht: Springer, 2007.

Bruckner, Donald W. "Considerations on the Morality of Meat Consumption: Hunted-Game versus Farm-Raised Animals." *Journal of Social Philosophy* 38.2 (2007): 311–30.

Brugger, E. Christian. "In Defense of Transferring Heterologous Embryos." *National Catholic Bioethics Quarterly* 5.1 (2005): 95–112.

Cahill, Lisa Sowle. "Catholicism, Death and Modern Medicine." *America.* April 25, 2005. http://www.bc.edu/bc_org/rvp/pubaf/04/AmericaOpEd Cahill0.html.

Cahoone, Lawrence. "Hunting as a Moral Good." *Environmental Values* 18.1 (2009): 67–89.

Capron, A. M. "The Bifurcated Legal Standard for Determining Death: Does It Work?" In *The Definition of Death: Contemporary Controversies,* edited by R. M. Arnold and R. Schapiro, 117–36. Baltimore: Johns Hopkins University Press, 1999.

Carlberg, Axel. "Transplanting Lungs from Non-Heart-Beating Donors." *National Catholic Bioethics Quarterly* 2.3 (2002): 377–80.

Cavagnaro, Charles E. "Treating Ectopic Pregnancy: A Moral Analysis (Part II)." *NaProEthics Forum* 4.2 (1999): 4.

Cavanaugh, Thomas. *Double Effect Reasoning: A Critique and Defense*. PhD diss., University of Notre Dame, 1995.

———. "The Intended/Foreseen Distinction's Ethical Relevance." *Philosophical Papers* 25.3 (1996): 179–88.

CDF (Congregation for the Doctrine of the Faith). *Dignitas Personae: Instruction on Certain Bioethical Questions*. Vatican City: Libreria Editrice Vaticana, 2008.

———. *Donum Vitae: Instruction on Respect for Human Life in Its Origin and on the Dignity of Procreation: Replies to Certain Questions of the Day*. Vatican City: Libreria Editrice Vaticana, 1987.

Chervenak, Frank A., and Laurence B. McCullough. "Ethics of Fetal Surgery." *Clinics in Perinatology* 36.2 (2009): 237–46.

Childress, James F. "Non-Heart-Beating Donors of Organs: Are the Distinctions between Direct and Indirect Effects and between Killing and Letting Die Relevant and Helpful?" *Kennedy Institute of Ethics Journal* 3.2 (1993): 203–16.

Chmaita, Ramen H., and Ruben A. Quintero. "Operative Fetoscopy in Complicated Monochorionic Twins: Current Status and Future Direction." *Current Opinion in Obstetrics and Gynecology* 20 (2008): 169–74.

Chopra, Anuj. "Childless Couples Look to India for Surrogate Mothers." *Christian Science Monitor,* April 3, 2006, http://www.csmonitor.com/2006/0403/p01s04-wosc.html.

Clark, Peter A. "Methotrexate and Tubal Pregnancies: Direct or Indirect Abortion?" *Linacre Quarterly* 67.1 (2000): 7–24.

———. "Tube Feedings and Persistent Vegetative State Patients: Ordinary or Extraordinary Means?" *Christian Bioethics* 12.1 (2006): 43–64.

Clark, Peter A., and Uday Deshmukh. "Non-Heart-Beating Organ Donation and Catholic Ethics." *National Catholic Bioethics Quarterly* 4.3 (2004): 537–51.

Cohen, Andrew I. "Contractarianism and Interspecies Welfare Conflicts." *Social Philosophy and Policy* 26.1 (2009): 227–57.

Connery, John. *Abortion: The Development of the Roman Catholic Perspective*. Chicago: Loyola University Press, 1977.

Cook, R. J., M. A. Olaya, and Bernard Dickens. "Healthcare Responsibilities and Conscientious Objection." *International Journal of Gynecology and Obstetrics* 104.3 (2009): 249–52.

Davis, Dena. "The Parental Investment Factor and the Child's Right to an Open Future." *Hastings Center Report* 39.2 (2009): 24–27.

Dekker, Teun. "The Illiberality of Perfectionist Enhancement." *Medicine, Health Care and Philosophy* 12.1 (2009): 91–98.

Delaney, Neil. "Two Cheers for 'Closeness': Terror, Targeting and Double Effect." *Philosophical Studies* 137.3 (2008): 335–67.

Dewan, Lawrence, OP. "St. Thomas, Rhonheimer, and the Moral Object." *Nova et Vetera English Edition* 6.1 (2008): 63–112.

Diamond, E. "Moral and Medical Considerations in the Management of Extrauterine Pregnancy." *Linacre Quarterly* 65 (1999): 5–45.

Dickens, Bernard. "Conscientious Objection and Professionalism." *Expert Reviews in Obstetrics and Gynecology* 4.2 (2009): 97–100.

———. "Conscientious Objection: A Shield or a Sword?" In *First Do No Harm: Law, Ethics, and Health Care,* edited by S. McLean, 337–51. Aldershot, England: Ashgate Publishing Group, 2006.

———. "Legal Protection and Limits of Conscientious Objection: When Conscientious Objection Is Unethical." *Medicine and Law* 28.2 (2009): 337–47.

Dixon, Ben. "Darwinism and Human Dignity." *Environmental Values* 16 (2007): 23–42.

Donagan, Alan. "Thomas Aquinas on Human Action." In *The Cambridge History of Later Medieval Philosophy,* edited by Norman Kretzmann, Anthony Kenny, and Jan Pinborg, 642–54. Cambridge: Cambridge University Press, 1982.

Drane, James F. "Stopping Nutrition and Hydration Technologies: A Conflict between Traditional Catholic Ethics and Church Authority." *Christian Bioethics* 12.1 (2006): 11–28.

DuBois, James M. "Avoiding Common Pitfalls in the Determination of Death." *National Catholic Bioethics Quarterly* 7.3 (2007): 545–60.

———. "Non-Heart-Beating Organ Donation: A Defense of the Required Determination of Death." *Journal of Law, Medicine & Ethics* 27.2 (1999): 126–36.

Dulles, Avery. "Religious Freedom: Innovation and Development." *First Things,* December 2001, 35–39.

Dworkin, Ronald, John Rawls, T. M. Scanlon, Robert Nozick, Thomas Nagel, and Judith Jarvis Thomson. "Assisted Suicide: The Philosophers' Brief." *New York Review of Books* 44.5 (1997): 41–47.

Eckert, E. D., T. J. Bouchard, J. Bohlen, and L. L. Heston. "Homosexuality in Monozygotic Twins Reared Apart." *British Journal of Psychiatry* 148 (1986): 421–25.

Engelhardt, H. Tristram. "Physician-Assisted Suicide: Dying as a Christian in a Post-Christian Age." *Christian Bioethics* 4.2 (1998): 143–67.

Finnis, John. *Aquinas: Moral, Political, and Legal Theory*. Founders of Modern Political and Social Thought. New York: Oxford University Press, 1998.

———. "Object and Intention in Moral Judgments according to Aquinas." *Thomist* 55.1 (1991): 1–27.

———. "The Rights and Wrongs of Abortion: A Reply to Judith Thomson." *Philosophy & Public Affairs* 2.2 (1973): 117–45.

Finnis, John, Germain Grisez, and Joseph Boyle. "'Direct' and 'Indirect': A Reply to Critics of Our Action Theory." *Thomist* 65.1 (2001): 1–44.

Flannery, Kevin L., SJ. "Aristotle and Human Movements." *Nova et Vetera English Edition* 6.1 (2008): 113–38.

Ford, John C., SJ. "The Morality of Obliteration Bombing." *Theological Studies* 5 (1944): 261–309.

Foster, Charles, Jonathan Herring, Karen Melham, and Tony Hope. "The Double Effect Effect." *Cambridge Quarterly of Healthcare Ethics* 20.1 (2011): 56–72.

Fuchs, Josef. "Gott—Der Herr über Leben und Tod." *Stimmen der Zeit* 214.121 (1996): 328–36.

Garcia, Jorge L. A. "A Catholic Perspective on the Ethics of Artificially Providing Food and Water." *Linacre Quarterly* 73.2 (2006): 132–52.

———. "The Doubling Undone? Double Effect in Recent Medical Ethics." *Philosophical Papers* 36.2 (2007): 245–70.

Gardiner, D., and B. Riley. "Non-Heart-Beating Organ Donation: Solution or a Step Too Far?" *Anaesthesia* 62.5 (2007): 431–33.

Gazzaniga, Michael S. "Humans: The Party Animal." *Daedalus* 138.3 (2009): 21–34.

Geach, Mary. "Are There Any Circumstances in Which It Would Be Morally Admirable for a Woman to Seek to Have an Orphan Embryo Implanted in Her Womb?" Paper presented at the Issues for a Catholic Bioethic Conference, Queens' College, Cambridge University, 1997.

Gelbaya, Tarek A. "Short- and Long-Term Risks to Women Who Conceive through In Vitro Fertilization." *Human Fertility* 13.1 (2010): 19–27.

George, Robert P., and Christopher Tollefsen. *Embryo: A Defense of Human Life*. New York: Doubleday, 2008.

Gerrard, J. W. "Is It Ethical for a General Practitioner to Claim a Conscientious Objection When Asked to Refer for Abortion?" *Journal of Medical Ethics* 35.10 (2009): 599–602.

Grall, T. S. "Support Providers: 2002. Household Economic Studies. Current Population Reports." Washington, DC: Bureau of the Census, 2007.

Grasser, Phyllis L. "Donation after Cardiac Death: Major Ethical Issues." *National Catholic Bioethics Quarterly* 7.3 (2007): 527–44.

Grisez, Germain. *Abortion: The Myths, the Realities, the Arguments*. New York: Corpus Books, 1970.

Gunnarsson, Logi. "The Great Apes and the Severely Disabled: Moral Status and Thick Evaluative Concepts." *Ethical Theory and Moral Practice* 11.3 (2008): 305–26.

Hansen, Michèle, Jennifer J. Kurinczuk, Carol Bower, and Sandra Webb. "The Risk of Major Birth Defects after Intracytoplasmic Sperm Injection and In Vitro Fertilization." *New England Journal of Medicine* 346.10 (2002): 725–30.

Harter, Thomas. "Overcoming the Organ Shortage: Failing Means and Radical Reform." *HEC Forum* 20.2 (2008): 155–82.

Harvey, John C. "The Burdens-Benefits Ratio Consideration for Medical Administration of Nutrition and Hydration to Persons in the Persistent Vegetative State." *Christian Bioethics* 12.1 (2006): 99–106.

Herdman, Roger, Thomas Beauchamp, and John T. Potts. "The Institute of Medicine's Report on Non-Heart-Beating Organ Transplantation." *Kennedy Institute of Ethics Journal* 8.1 (1998): 83–90.

Hills, Alison. "Intentions, Foreseen Consequences and the Doctrine of Double Effect." *Philosophical Studies* 133.2 (2007): 257–83.

Hitti, Miranda. "CDC: IVF May Boost Birth Defect Risk." *WebMD Health News*. November 17, 2008. http://www.webmd.com/infertility-and-reproduction/news/20081117/cdc-ivf-may-boost-birth-defects-risk.

Hobbes, Thomas. *The English Works of Thomas Hobbes of Malmesbury*. London: John Bohn, 1839–1845.

Hopkins, Patrick D. "Can Technology Fix the Abortion Problem? Ectogenesis and the Real Issues of Abortion." *International Journal of Applied Philosophy* 22.2 (2008): 311–26.

Howsepian, A. A. . "On Referring." *Ethics and Medicine* 25.1 (2009): 31–47.

Hursthouse, Rosalind. *Beginning Lives*. Oxford: Oxford University Press, 1987.

Jamieson, Dale. "The Rights of Animals and the Demands of Nature." *Environmental Values* 17.2 (2008): 181–99.

Jensen, Steven J. "Getting Inside the Acting Person." *International Philosophical Quarterly* 50.4 (2010): 461–71.

———. *Good and Evil Actions: A Journey through Saint Thomas Aquinas*. Washington, DC: Catholic University of America Press, 2010.

John Paul II, Pope. *Evangelium Vitae*. Vatican City: Libreria Editrice Vaticana, 1995.

———. "If You Want Peace, Respect the Conscience of Every Person." Message for the 1991 World Day of Peace. *Acta Apostolicae Sedis* 83 (1991): 414–15.

———. *Tertio Mellenio.* Vatican City: Libreria Editrice Vaticana, 1997.

———. *Veritatis Splendor.* Vatican City: Libreria Editrice Vaticana, 1993.

Kaczor, Christopher. "Capital Punishment and the Catholic Tradition: Contradiction, Change in Circumstance, or Development of Doctrine." *Nova et Vetera English Edition* 2.1 (2004): 279–304.

———. "Distinguishing Intention from Foresight: What Is Included in a Means to an End?" *International Philosophical Quarterly* 41.1 (2001): 77–89.

———. "Double-Effect Reasoning: From Jean Pierre Gury to Peter Knauer." *Theological Studies* 59 (1998): 297–316.

———. *The Edge of Life: Human Dignity and Contemporary Bioethics.* Philosophy and Medicine. Dordrecht: Springer, 2005.

———. "Equal Rights, Unequal Wrongs." *First Things,* August–September 2011, 21–23.

———. *The Ethics of Abortion: Women's Rights, Human Life, and the Question of Justice.* Routledge Annals of Bioethics. New York: Routledge, 2011.

———. "Intention, Foresight, and Mutilation: A Response to Giebel." *International Philosophical Quarterly* 47.4 (2007): 481–86.

Kain, Patrick. "Kant's Defense of Human Moral Status." *Journal of the History of Philosophy* 47.1 (2009): 59–102.

Kamm, Frances M. "The Doctrine of Triple Effect and Why a Rational Agent Need Not Intend the Means to His End." *Aristotelian Society Supplementary Volume* 74.1 (2000): 21–39.

Kant, Immanuel. *Grounding for the Metaphysics of Morals.* Translated by James E. Ellington. Indianapolis: Hackett, 1993.

———. *Grundlegung zur Metaphysik der Sitten.* Edited by Wilhelm Weischedel. Wiesbaden: Insel Verlag, 1956.

Keown, John. *Euthanasia, Ethics and Public Policy: An Argument against Legalisation.* Cambridge: Cambridge University Press, 2002.

———. "The Legal Revolution: From 'Sanctity of Life' to 'Quality of Life' and 'Autonomy.'" In *Issues for a Catholic Bioethic,* edited by Luke Gormally, 233–60. London: Linacre Center, 1999.

Keown, John, and David Jones. "Surveying the Foundations of Medical Law: A Reassessment of Glanville Williams's *The Sanctity of Life and the Criminal Law.*" *Medical Law Review* 16.1 (2008): 85–126.

Kissling, Frances. "Abortion Rights Are under Attack, and Pro-Choice Advocates Are Caught in a Time Warp." *The Washington Post.* February 18, 2011. http:

//www.washingtonpost.com/wp-dyn/content/article/2011/02/18/AR2011
021802434.html.

Kittay, Eva Feder. "The Personal Is Philosophical Is Political: A Philosopher and
Mother of a Cognitively Disabled Person Sends Notes from the Battlefield."
Metaphilosophy 40.3–4 (2009): 606–27.

Knapp, Christopher. "Species Inegalitarianism as a Matter of Principle." *Journal
of Applied Philosophy* 26.2 (2009): 174–89.

Kootstra, G., J. H. C. Daemen, and A. P. A. Oomen. "Categories of Non-Heart-
Beating Donors." *Transplantation Proceedings* 27.5 (1995): 2893–94.

Koren, Gideon. "Adverse Effects of Assisted Reproductive Technology and
Pregnancy Outcome: A Review Of: Stromberg B, Dahlquist LG, Ericson
A, et al. 2002. Teratological Sequelae in Children Born after in Vitro Fer-
tilization: A Population Based Study. Lancet 359: 461–465; Schieve LA,
Meikle SF, Ferre C, et al. 2002. Low and Very Low Birth Weight in Infants
Conceived with Use of Assisted Reproductive Technology. N Engl J Med
346: 731–737; and Hansen M, Kurnczuk JJ, Bower C, et al. 2002. The
Risk of Major Birth Defects after Intracytoplasmic Sperm Injection and in
Vitro Fertilization. N Engl J Med 346:725–730." *Pediatric Research* 52.2
(2002): 136.

Leach, C. L., et al. "Partial Liquid Ventilation with Perflubron in Premature Infants with Severe Respiratory Distress Syndrome." *New England Journal of
Medicine* 335 (1996): 761–67.

Lee, Patrick. *Abortion and Unborn Human Life*. Washington, DC: Catholic University of America Press, 1996.

Lee, Patrick, and Robert P. George. *Body-Self Dualism in Contemporary Ethics and
Politics*. New York: Cambridge University Press, 2007.

Levin, Yuval. "Indignity and Bioethics: Steven Pinker Discovers the Human-
Dignity Cabal." *National Review Online*. May 14, 2008. http://article
.nationalreview.com/?q=NmNiY2UyYzUwNDE1ODIxNWQ0YzFhYWFi
ZmRmYjVhMmQ.

Lewis, C. S. *The Abolition of Man*. New York: Macmillan, 1955.

Liao, S. Matthew. "The Basis of Human Moral Status." *Journal of Moral Philosophy* 7.2 (2010): 159–79.

———. "The Loop Case and Kamm's Doctrine of Triple Effect." *Philosophical
Studies* 146.2 (2009): 223–31.

Locke, John. *The Second Treatise on Government*. Indianapolis: Hackett, 1980.

Long, Stephen A. "*Veritatis Splendor* §78 and the Moral Act." *Nova et Vetera English Edition* 6.1 (2008): 139–56.

Manninen, Bertha Alvarez. "Rethinking *Roe v. Wade:* Defending the Abortion Right in the Face of Contemporary Opposition." *American Journal of Bioethics* 10.12 (2010): 33–46.

Marquis, Don. "Manninen's Defense of Abortion Rights Is Unsuccessful." *American Journal of Bioethics* 10.12 (2010): 56–57.

———. "Review of Christopher Kaczor, *The Ethics of Abortion: Women's Rights, Human Life, and the Question of Justice.*" *Notre Dame Philosophical Reviews.* November 10, 2010. http://ndpr.nd.edu/news/24538-the-ethics-of-abortion-women-s-rights-human-life-and-the-question-of-justice/.

———. "Why Abortion Is Immoral." In *Bioethics: An Anthology,* edited by Helga Kuhse and Peter Singer. Malden, MA: Blackwell, 1999.

Masek, Lawrence. "Intentions, Motives and the Doctrine of Double Effect." *Philosophical Quarterly* 60.240 (2010): 567–85.

Mattox, M. Casey, and Matthew S. Bowman. "Your Conscience, Your Right: A History of Efforts to Violate Pro-Life Medical Conscience, and the Laws That Stand in the Way." *Linacre Quarterly* 77.2 (2010): 187–97.

May, Thomas, and Mark P. Aulisio. "Personal Morality and Professional Obligations: Rights of Conscience and Informed Consent." *Perspectives in Biology and Medicine* 52.1 (2009): 30–38.

May, William E. "Caring for Persons in the 'Persistent Vegetative State' and Pope John Paul II's March 20, 2004, Address 'On Life-Sustaining Treatments and the Vegetative State.'" *Medicina e Morale* 55 (2005): 533–55.

———. *Catholic Bioethics and the Gift of Human Life.* 2nd ed. Huntingdon, IN: Our Sunday Visitor Publishing, 2008.

———. "The Management of Ectopic Pregnancies: A Moral Analysis." In *The Fetal Tissue Issue: Medical and Ethical Aspects,* edited by Peter J. Cataldo and Albert S. Moraczewski, OP, 121–48. Braintree, MA: Pope John Center, 1994.

———. "Methotrexate and Ectopic Pregnancy." *Ethics & Medics* 23.3 (1998): 1–3.

McCullough, Laurence B., and Frank A. Chervenak. *Ethics in Obstetrics and Gynecology.* New York: Oxford University Press, 1994.

McInerny, Ralph. *Aquinas on Human Action: A Theory of Practice.* Washington, DC: Catholic University of America Press, 1992.

McMahan, Jeff. "Eating Animals the Nice Way." *Daedalus* 137.1 (2008): 66–76.

Mill, John Stuart. *Utilitarianism.* Indianapolis: Hackett, 1979.

Miller, Franklin G., and Robert D. Truog. "The Incoherence of Determining Death by Neurological Criteria: A Commentary on *Controversies in the Determination of Death,* a White Paper by the President's Council on Bioethics." *Kennedy Institute of Ethics Journal* 19.2 (2009): 185–93.

Moir, Anne, and David Jessel. *Brain Sex: The Real Difference between Men and Women.* New York: Delta, 1991.

Moraczewski, Albert. "Managing Tubal Pregnancies: Part 1." *Ethics & Medics* 21.6 (1996): 1–3.

———. "Managing Tubal Pregnancies: Part 2." *Ethics & Medics* 21.8 (1996): 3–4.

Morlock, R. J., et al. "Cost-Effectiveness of Single-Dose Methotrexate Compared with Laparoscopic Treatment of Ectopic Pregnancy." *Obstetrics and Gynecology* 95.3 (2000): 407–12.

Mullady, Brian. "Religious Liberty: Homogeneous or Heterogeneous Development?" *Thomist* 58.1 (1994): 93–108.

Murphy, Timothy F. "Choosing Disabilities and Enhancements in Children: A Choice Too Far?" *Reproductive Medicine Online* 18.S1 (2009): S43–S49.

———. "The Ethics of Helping Transgender Men and Women Have Children." *Perspectives in Biology and Medicine* 53.1 (2010): 46–60.

National Conference of Commissioners on Uniform State Laws. Uniform Determination of Death Act, 1980. Chicago: n.p., 1980.

Neuhaus, Richard John. *The Naked Public Square: Religion and Democracy in America.* 2nd ed. Grand Rapids, MI: Eerdmans, 1986.

New York Times. "400,000 Embryos and Counting." Editorial. May 15, 2003.

Noonan, John T. *Contraception: A History of Its Treatment by the Catholic Theologians and Canonists.* Cambridge, MA: Harvard University Press, 1986.

O'Brien, Dennis. "Can We Talk about Abortion?" *Commonweal.* September 12, 2011. http://commonwealmagazine.org/print/5968.

Oderberg, David. *Applied Ethics: A Non-Consequentialist Approach.* Oxford: Blackwell, 2000.

O'Rourke, Kevin. "Reflections on the Papal Allocution Concerning Care for Persistent Vegetative State Patients." *Christian Bioethics* 12.1 (2006): 83–97.

Orr, Robert D. "Ethics and Life's Ending." *First Things,* August–September 2004, 31–35.

———. "Medical Ethics and the Faith Factor: The Endangered Right of Conscience." *Ethics & Medicine* 26.1 (2010): 49–54.

Ott, Ludwig. *Fundamentals of Catholic Dogma.* Translated by Patrick Lynch. Rockford, IL: TAN Books, 1974.

Pacholczyk, Tad. "Some Moral Contraindications to Embryo Adoption." In *The Ethics of Embryo Adoption and the Catholic Tradition,* edited by Sarah-Vaughan Brakman and Darlene Fozard Weaver, 69–84. Dordrecht: Springer, 2007.

Padawer, Ruth. "The Two-Minus-One Pregnancy." *The New York Times Magazine,* August 10, 2011. http://www.nytimes.com/2011/08/14/magazine/the-two-minus-one-pregnancy.html?pagewanted=all.

Parents Involved in Community Schools v. Seattle School District No. 1. 551 U.S. 701 (2007).

Pascal, Blaise. *Oeuvres Complètes.* Edited by Louis LaFuma. Paris: Aux Éditions due Deuil, 1963.

Pellegrino, Edmund D., Adam Schulman, and Thomas W. Merrill, eds. *Human Dignity and Bioethics.* Washington, DC: U.S. Independent Agencies and Commissions, 2008.

Pinckaers, Servais. *Somme Théologique: Les Actes Humaines.* Vol. 1. Paris: Desclée, 1962.

Pinker, Steven. "The Stupidity of Dignity: Conservative Bioethics' Latest, Most Dangerous Ploy." *New Republic,* May 28, 2008, 28–31.

Plantinga, Alvin. *Warrant and Proper Function.* New York: Oxford University Press, 1993.

Popenoe, David, and Barbara Dafoe Whitehead. "Should We Live Together? What Young Adults Need to Know About Cohabitation before Marriage: A Comprehensive Review of Recent Research." Rutgers, NJ: National Marriage Project, 2002.

Porter, Maureen, Valerie Peddie, and Siladitya Bhattacharya. "Debate: Do Upper Age Limits Need to Be Imposed on Women Receiving Assisted Reproduction Treatment?" *Human Fertility* 10.2 (2007): 87–92.

Prusak, Bernard G. "Breaking the Bond: Abortion and the Grounds of Parental Obligations." *Social Theory and Practice* 37.2 (2011): 311–32.

———. "What Are Parents For?" *Hastings Center Report* 40.2 (2010): 37–47.

Quinn, Warren. "Actions, Intentions, and Consequences: The Doctrine of Double Effect." *Philosophy and Public Affairs* 18.4 (1989): 334–51.

Rajczi, Alex. "Abortion, Competing Entitlements, and Parental Responsibility." *Journal of Applied Philosophy* 26.4 (2009): 379–95.

Regnerus, Mark. "How Different Are the Adult Children of Parents Who Have Same-Sex Relationships? Findings from the New Family Structures Study." *Social Science Research* 41.4 (2012): 752–70.

Reichmann, James. *Evolution, Animal "Rights," and the Environment.* Washington, DC: Catholic University of America Press, 2000.

Rhoads, Steven E. *Taking Sex Differences Seriously.* New York: Encounter Books, 2005.

Rhonheimer, Martin. *The Perspective of the Acting Person: Essays in the Renewal of Thomistic Moral Philosophy.* Edited by William F. Murphy, Jr. Washington DC: Catholic University of America Press, 2008.

———. "The Truth About Condoms." *The Tablet,* July 10, 2004, 10–11.

Robertson, John A. "The Octuplet Case—Why More Regulation Is Not Likely." *Hastings Center Report* 39.3 (2009): 26–28.

Rock, John. *Telinde's Operative Gynecology*. Philadelphia: Lippincott-Raven, 1992.

Rossi, A. Cristina, and Vincenzo D'Addario. "Umbilical Cord Occlusion for Selective Feticide in Complicated Monochorionic Twins: A Systematic Review of Literature." *American Journal of Obstetrics and Gynecology* 200.2 (2009): 123–29.

Saletan, William. "Half-Aborted: Why Do 'Reductions' of Twin Pregnancies Trouble Pro-Choicers?" *Slate,* August 16, 2011. http://www.slate.com/id /2301322/.

Salon, J. E. "Perflubron in Infants with Severe Respiratory Distress Syndrome." *New England Journal of Medicine* 336 (1997): 660.

Savulescu, Julian, and Guy Kahane. "The Moral Obligation to Create Children with the Best Chance of the Best Life." *Bioethics* 23.5 (2008): 274–90.

Sax, Leonard. *Why Gender Matters*. New York: Broadway, 2006.

Schmidt, Lone. "Should Men and Women Be Encouraged to Start Childbearing at a Younger Age?" *Expert Review of Obstetrics and Gynecology* 5.2 (2010): 145–48.

Second Vatican Council. *Lumen Gentium* (Dogmatic Constitution on the Church). November 21, 1964. http://www.vatican.va/archive/hist_councils/ ii_vatican_council/documents/vat-ii_const_19641121_lumen-gentium_ en.html.

Sepilian, Vicken, and Ellen Wood. "Ectopic Pregnancy." *Medscape Reference.* Updated August 2, 2012. http://emedicine.medscape.com/article/2041923 -overview.

Shannon, Thomas A. "Nutrition and Hydration: An Analysis of the Recent Papal Statement in Light of the Roman Catholic Bioethical Tradition." *Christian Bioethics* 12.1 (2006): 29–41.

Shettles, L. "Tubal Embryo Successfully Transplanted in Utero." *American Journal of Obstetrics and Gynecology* 163.6 (1990): 2026–27.

Shewmon, D. Alan. "The Brain and Somatic Integration: Insights into the Standard Biological Rationale for Equating 'Brain Death' with Death." *Journal of Medicine and Philosophy* 26.5 (2001): 475–78.

———. "Brain Death: Can It Be Resuscitated?" *Hastings Center Report* 39.2 (2009): 18–24.

———. "Brainstem Death, Brain Death, and Death: A Critical Re-Evaluation." *Issues in Law & Medicine* 14.2 (1998): 125–45.

———. "The Dead Donor Rule: Lessons from Linguistics?" *Kennedy Institute of Ethics Journal* 14.3 (2004): 277–300.

Singer, Peter. "Famine, Affluence, and Morality." In *What's Wrong? Applied Ethicists and Their Critics,* edited by David Boonin and Graham Oddie, 537–44. Oxford: Oxford University Press, 2005.

————. "Speciesism and Moral Status." *Metaphilosophy* 40.3–4 (2009): 567–81.

Singer, Peter, and Deane Wells. *The Reproduction Revolution: New Ways of Making Babies.* Oxford: Oxford University Press, 1984.

Smajdor, Anna. "Should IVF Guidelines Be Relaxed in the UK?" *Expert Review of Obstetrics & Gynecology* 4.5 (2009): 501–8.

Smith, Janet E., and Christopher Kaczor. *Life Issues, Medical Choices.* Cincinnati, OH: Servant Books, 2007.

Smith, William B. "Rescue the Frozen?" *Homiletic and Pastoral Review* 96.1 (1996): 72–74.

Spielthenner, Georg. "The Principle of Double Effect as a Guide for Medical Decision-Making." *Medicine, Health Care and Philosophy* 11.4 (2008): 465–73.

Sprigg, Peter, and Timothy Dailey. *Getting It Straight: What the Research Shows About Homosexuality.* Washington, DC: Family Research Council, 2004.

Stacey, Judith, and Timothy J. Biblarz. "(How) Does the Sexual Orientation of Parents Matter?" *American Sociological Review* 66.2 (2001): 159–83.

Stanford University School of Medicine. "Deceased Donor as a Source of Organs for Heart Transplantation." Ashley Lab, Stanford University School of Medicine, 2013. http://ashleylab.stanford.edu/projects/physclin/non_heart_beat _donor.html.

Stanmeyer, John. "An Embryo Adoptive Father's Perspective." In *The Ethics of Embryo Adoption and the Catholic Tradition,* edited by Sarah-Vaughan Brakman and Darlene Fozard Weaver, 231–50. Dordrecht: Springer, 2007.

Steinberg, David. "The Antemortem Use of Heparin in Non-Heart-Beating Organ Transplantation: A Justification Based on the Paradigm of Altruism." *Journal of Clinical Ethics* 14.1–2 (2003): 18–25.

Strömberg, B., G. Dahlquist, O. Finnstrom, M. Koster, K. Stjernqvist, and A. Ericson. "Neurological Sequelae in Children Born after In-Vitro Fertilisation: A Population-Based Study." *Lancet* 359.9305 (2002): 461.

Sulmasy, Daniel. "Dignity and Bioethics: History, Theory, and Selected Applications." In *Human Dignity and Bioethics,* edited by Adam Schulman, Edmund D. Pellegrino, and Thomas W. Merrill, 469–501. Washington, DC: U.S. Independent Agencies and Commissions, 2008.

Thomasma, David. "Assisted Death and Martyrdom." *Christian Bioethics* 4.2 (1998): 122–42.

Tonti-Filippini, Nicholas. "The Embryo Rescue Debate: Impregnating Women, Ectogenesis, and Restoration from Suspended Animation." *National Catholic Bioethics Quarterly* 3.1 (2003): 111–37.

Tuohey, John F. "The Implications of the *Ethical and Religious Directives for Catholic Health Services* on the Clinical Practice of Resolving the Ectopic Pregnancy." *Louvain Studies* 20 (1995): 41–57.

United Nations General Assembly. *Universal Declaration of Human Rights.* GA res. 217 A (III). December 10, 1948. http://www.un.org/en/documents/udhr/.

United States Conference of Catholic Bishops (USCCB). "The Catholic Church in America—Meeting Real Needs in Your Neighborhood." Catholic Information Project. 2006. http://nccbuscc.org/comm/2006CIPFinal.pdf.

————. *Ethical and Religious Directives for Catholic Health Care Services.* 4th ed. Washington, DC: USCCB Publishing Services, 2001.

University of Pittsburgh. "University of Pittsburgh Medical Center Policy and Procedure Manual." *Kennedy Institute of Ethics Journal* 3.2 (1993): A1–A15.

Ursin, Lars Øystein. "Personal Autonomy and Informed Consent." *Medicine, Health Care and Philosophy* 12.1 (2009): 17–24.

Valko, Nancy. "Ethical Implications of Non-Heart-Beating Organ Donation." *Human Life Review* 28.3 (2002): 107–12.

Varelius, Jukka. "Minimally Conscious State and Human Dignity " *Neuroethics* 2.1 (2009): 35–50.

Verheijde, J. L., M. Y. Rady, and J. McGregor. "Recovery of Transplantable Organs after Cardiac or Circulatory Death: Transforming the Paradigm for the Ethics of Organ Donation." *Philosophy, Ethics, and Humanities in Medicine* 2.8 (2007): 1–8.

Ville, Yves. "Fetal Therapy: Practical Ethical Considerations." *Prenatal Diagnosis* 31.7 (2011): 621–27.

Waldron, Jeremy. "Dignity, Rank, and Rights." 2009 Tanner Lectures at UC Berkeley. NYU School of Law, Public Law Research Paper No. 09-50. http://ssrn.com/abstract=1461220.

Wallace, C. J. "Transplantation of Ectopic Pregnancy from Fallopian Tube to Cavity of Uterus." *Surgery, Gynecology, and Obstetrics* 24 (1917): 578–79.

Walters, Patrick, and Maryclaire Dale. "DA: West Philadelphia Abortion Doctor Killed 7 Babies with Scissors." WPVI-TV. January 21, 2011. http://abclocal.go.com/wpvi/story?section=news/local&id=7906881.

Wardle, Lynn. "The Potential Impact of Homosexual Parenting on Children." *University of Illinois Law Review* (1997): 833–919.

Westberg, Daniel. "Aquinas and the Process of Human Action." In *Moral and Political Philosophy in the Middle Ages: Proceedings of the Ninth International Congress of Medieval Philosophy,* edited by B. Bazán, E. Andújar, and L. Sbrocchi, 816–25. Ottawa: Legas, 1992.

————. *Right Practical Reason. Aristotle, Action, and Prudence in Aquinas.* Oxford: Clarendon Press, 1994.

White, Alan. *Grounds of Liability: An Introduction to the Philosophy of Law.* Oxford: Clarendon Press, 1985.

Wicclair, Mark R. "Conscience-Based Exemptions for Medical Students." *Cambridge Quarterly of Health Care Ethics* 19.1 (2010): 38–50.

———. "Is Conscientious Objection Incompatible with a Physician's Professional Obligations?" *Theoretical Medicine and Bioethics* 29.3 (2008): 171–85.

Wilcox, W. Bradford, William Doherty, Norval Glenn, and Linda Waite. "Why Marriage Matters: Twenty-Six Conclusions from the Social Sciences." New York: Institute for American Values, 2005.

Williams, Bernard, and J. J. C. Smart. *Utilitarianism: For and Against.* Cambridge: Cambridge University Press, 1973.

Zeiler, K., E. Furberg, G. Tufveson, and S. Welin. "The Ethics of Non-Heart-Beating Donation: How New Technology Can Change the Ethical Landscape." *Journal of Medical Ethics* 34.7 (2008): 526–29.

Zimmerman, Sacha. "Ectogenesis: Development of Artificial Wombs." *San Francisco Chronicle,* Sunday, August 24, 2003, D3.

———. "The Fetal Position: The Real Threat to *Roe v. Wade.*" *New Republic,* August 18, 2003, 14–17.

Index

Christopher Kaczor

is professor of philosophy at Loyola Marymount University in Los Angeles.

He is author and editor of a number of books,

including *The Ethics of Abortion:*

Women's Rights, Human Life, and the Question of Justice